INTERGENERATIONAL

Intergenerational

How Sickness and Health
Take Root in Families, Organizations,
and Relationships

LAUREN VIGNEC

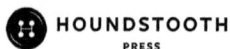

HOUNDSTOOTH
PRESS

INTERGENERATIONAL
How Sickness and Health Take Root in Families,
Organizations, and Relationships

FIRST EDITION

ISBN   978-1-5445-4542-4   *Paperback*
        978-1-5445-4543-1   *Ebook*

CONTENTS

INTRODUCTION

AS WE HEAD TO THE LAS VEGAS AIRPORT, I MENTION to my seventy-year-old rideshare driver that I am a pastor.

Turns out he was also a pastor. Retired now, but he worshiped in the Baptist Church his whole life. Married for more than forty years, but his wife didn't come to God until age thirty-five. She was in a singing trio, like the Supremes. Apparently, they toured all over. I guess they got pretty big in California before having to call it quits.

The conversation keeps wandering. I talk about being a financial advisor, calling it "my career that actually pays. Being a pastor doesn't pay." He laughs and agrees. He describes learning Scripture by listening to books on tape while driving eighteen-wheelers for a living.

He mentions his life now being filled with joy, and that a big part of that joy is working—staying busy. He is retired, but not really retired. I say, "No one ever really retires nowadays." He thinks that's pretty funny too.

Then our conversation shifts. He talks about how his job

now is to plant a seed, "and you will receive a harvest. You can't tell other people what to do." The moment he mentions not telling other people what to do, my ears and the hair on my arms prick up.

He talks about how so many people are broken and how other people he meets are consumed by bitterness, even for someone long dead.

I think about his statement: *You can't tell other people what to do.* I tell him, "You are exactly right about that."

I start talking about an alcoholic friend of mine. I say, "Here's me." I point to myself. "Here's my friend." I point to the dash. "And here's my friend's drinking." I point to the window.

"I can affect my relationship to my friend." I trace a line from me to the dash. "And I can even affect my own relationship to my friend's drinking. For instance, I can tell him I just won't hang out with him when he drinks." I trace a line from me to the window. "But I can't affect his relationship to his drinking!" I trace a line from the dash to the window.

"I can never make someone else more responsible. Anything I do to try to make him more responsible for his drinking causes *me* to take some responsibility for *his* drinking. And that means now he has even *less* responsibility."

Chuckling, the driver agrees. "Because now all he has to do is call you up and unload it all on you!"

"Yes," he says, "you have to love people where they are at. I never try to fix or save anyone. I just pray that God will give me a word to give people—to plant that seed."

I say, "That is right! I can't act like I'm someone's father. Because then they act toward me based on where I'm at in their own emotional family tree. And speaking of bitterness toward someone long dead, well, if I start to act like someone's father..."

We arrive at the airport. The driver says, "I don't take anything lightly. There is a reason we needed to meet."

As we shake hands, we both say the same phrase at the same time: "Take care of yourself."

Most people just say, "Take care." They don't use the whole phrase. We both did, and we both meant it.

It's funny because I had been struggling for years to figure out the simplest way to explain concepts about boundaries and responsibility that transformed the way I work and live. Then, in an eight-minute conversation, a Las Vegas Lyft driver gave me the perfect example:

Because now all he has to do is call you up and unload it all on you!

* * *

The Lyft driver had hoped our conversation would plant a seed, and my hope is that this book does the same. This is the book I wish I could have read when I started out as a pastor. This was the book I needed.

I never intended to join the clergy, by the way. In fact, I avoided that calling for years because I didn't want to follow in my father's footsteps.

See, my father was not just a pastor. He was a truly beloved one in the city of Tacoma, Washington. When he passed away, his funeral was featured on the front page of the local paper.

Everyone seemed to know him, from the mayor to the local gangsters who would ask me, "How does it feel to have a father who is famous? Your dad is the president of Tacoma!" They were saying this about a preacher who never even had a church building, a man who always figured out a way to convince someone to offer a rent-free space to worship.

My father was not only charismatic but also unusual and unpredictable, a maverick. He had started a church in the Salishan projects, which was a low-income development originally intended as temporary housing for soldiers during World War II. His mission was to serve those experiencing poverty, but soon the congregation attracted all kinds of folks who only had one thing in common: none felt welcomed at a regular church.

This made for some surprising experiences for me as a pastor's kid. I remember when the gangs moved up from Los Angeles, and Tacoma was not ready for them. Many of my friends started wearing those colors, identified as members, and began a whole new life that I could perceive but never participate in. They still came to our church though, and we remained friends through gunshot wounds, arrests, and prison stints.

By the time I became the church's pastor, everything had changed. For one, the community was no longer exclusively low-income. Second, the church's mission had become more focused on ex-convicts and their families. I started doing prison ministry as well. Now, I'm not making any comment here about whether or not the people in prison ought to be there. But the blunt reality is that incarceration focuses on those who have experienced poverty, mental illness, addiction, and domestic violence. So, in my role as a pastor, those are the issues I deal with.

And speaking of mental illness, I connect well with my congregation members partly because of my personal experience. I have always had hallucinations, and for a long time my life was consumed by my battle with clinical depression and delusion. I refer to the worst period, which lasted from about age twenty to age thirty-five, as my "lost years." I often tell people I have no idea what it's like to be inside a prison, but I do know what it's like to want fifteen years of my life back.

I also became a financial advisor, which might not seem to be the sort of career that fits with prison ministry. Well, my father had one sister, and she owned a financial services business. So aside from inheriting my father's role, I also went to work for my aunt. She taught me, among other things, how to be an entrepreneur.

In 2009 I started my own business. By around 2016 or so I achieved financial independence. That sounds like an easy story, but it leaves out the nightmares I had when I began. I was terrified of failing because, in my first year, I straight up lost money. I was paying more to rent my office than I was making in fees. I figured out that I'd better quickly find a way to get clients or else I wasn't going to eat, so I started preparing tax returns.

A large proportion of the folks who are willing to pay for tax preparation are small business owners, so I got to know all kinds of entrepreneurs, shop owners, plumbers, and side-hustlers. As a result, I started doing business consulting. And I did eventually thrive as a financial advisor, so yes, I work with some wealthy folks. But I also spend a lot of time with retired middle-class people talking about the arc of their lives—the trajectory of their marriages and families.

As a result of my multiple careers, I have a genuine, concrete connection with the day-to-day financial experiences of just about the whole range of American society, from the very poor to the very rich. I have broad experience working with every kind of family, from the happiest to the most dysfunctional. I've worked with all kinds of relationships and marriages, and with a fascinating collection of businesses and other organizations.

I've made mistakes as a pastor, as a business consultant, and as a financial advisor. And a few years ago I realized my mistakes had a common source. It wasn't just that I was screwing up. My worldview, my entire perspective, was flawed. In fact, in some ways it was backwards. I had to learn a whole new way of thinking.

I look around and I see so many people making the same kinds of mistakes I made. These are people who are committed, genuine, and compassionate, but they suffer under the same misguided worldview I used to hold. If you are someone who wants to heal sick families, dysfunctional organizations, or toxic relationships, this book is for you.

Very few ideas in this book represent my own innovations. They come from micro-sociology and family systems theory, which is discussed among some sociologists, psychiatrists, and clergy, but not well known outside those circles. So the ideas are already out there floating around, but they are not easily accessible.

I hope this book makes what I had to learn accessible. I hope it popularizes a way of thinking about human interaction that, while opposed to much current conventional wisdom, was probably familiar to your ancestors. And maybe it will allow you to avoid the mistakes I made, while helping you to start, grow, and maintain healthy families, organizations, and relationships.

This book is a seed, and I hope it comes to you as a good word.

Table of Contents
Chapter 1: The Family Is Sick; the Individual Shows Symptoms

I believe that especially when it comes to mental illness, gut health, and behavioral issues, many disorders and conditions are just symptoms. The real sickness is often in the family itself, not in any particular individual. The word "family" here refers to any group of people who have strong emotional connections with one another, so the same individual can also be showing symptoms from more than one family. No one will heal as long as the focus stays on the individual, in part because the sickest member of any family is usually not the one showing the worst symptoms.

Chapter 2: The Family's Response to Its Own Sickness

The family's response to individual symptoms can be even worse than the symptoms themselves. The family member with the most severe or most attention-grabbing symptoms often gets "diagnosed" or labeled, almost becoming a scapegoat. Once an individual's symptoms are diagnosed as a medical problem, a mental health issue, or a personality disorder, the family sickness itself is ignored. So even if a symptom gets "fixed" in one individual, it just pops up somewhere else in the family as a new symptom.

Chapter 3: How to Start Healing a Sick Family

Fortunately, healing a sick family does not require the ability to perfectly distinguish between sickness, symptoms, and response to symptoms. Instead, healing starts whenever any family member, regardless of position or status, stops participating in the cycle of sickness. You can start the healing process by staying connected to the other family members while refusing to take sides in their conflicts with each other.

Chapter 4: Why Do So Many of Us Seem to Recreate Our Family's Sickness?

Healing is difficult, though, because we carry around our family dynamics and memories in our heads. This is how we "talk to ourselves," "take care of ourselves," and, occasionally, "lie to ourselves." Since we carry our families with us, we also carry predetermined and prejudged ideas about our relationships with others. When we meet new people, we often recreate the family trauma we are used to without even realizing what we're doing.

Chapter 5: How Sickness and Health Become Intergenerational

No matter what your intentions, whenever you do not deal with sickness in any family—and your own participation in it— you pass that sickness on to the next family you are involved in. So does every other human being you interact with. This is the process by which sickness becomes intergenerational. Many symptoms you suffer from may be coming from someone you barely remember or never even met.

Chapter 6: The Role You Play Matters More than You Think It Does

People react not to you but to your perceived role in the family. That role is a mix of the actual family role you play and whatever memories and ideas people project onto you. You also do the same to everyone around you. We live not in a world of interacting individuals but also in a world of interlocking relationships—connected families.

Chapter 7: Emotional Energy

It is almost as if our minds exist in emotional fields the way objects exist in gravitational fields. And our habitual interactions with others, our daily rituals, produce those emotional fields. Through these rituals, many of which are also intergenerational, we create the emotional energy and well-being that invigorate healthy families.

Chapter 8: How to Transform Your Emotional Reality

In a healthy family, you can accelerate the long process of intergenerational health by changing your emotional habits. You can redefine what it means to "win" and turn even your most negative emotions into powerful allies.

Chapter 9: Radical Responsibility and Intergenerational Health

As your emotional responses change, you will see the world more clearly. True clarity comes when you realize you are 100 percent responsible for your relationship to any other person, and you are 0 percent responsible for anyone's relationship to anyone else. You are also 100 percent responsible for your relationship to any idea, goal or issue, and 0 percent responsible for anyone else's relationship to anything else. The daily practice of radical responsibility will heal and revitalize your families, organizations, and relationships.

CHAPTER 1

THE FAMILY IS SICK

The Individual Shows Symptoms

I believe that especially when it comes to mental illness, gut health, and behavioral issues, many disorders and conditions are just symptoms. The real sickness is often in the family itself, not in any particular individual. The word "family" here refers to any group of people who have strong emotional connections with one another, so the same individual can also be showing symptoms from more than one family. No one will heal as long as the focus stays on the individual, in part because the sickest member of any family is usually not the one showing the worst symptoms.

WHEN I HAVE A HEADACHE, THE SYMPTOM IS THAT MY head hurts. But the actual problem is usually somewhere else— my back or my feet, generally. In fact the problem might not even be physical. It could be stress, for instance.

Similarly, a member of a family ("family" meaning any

emotionally connected group) may show symptoms of depression, eating disorders, sexual acting-out, rage, paranoia, anxiety, alcoholism, drug abuse, stomachaches, headaches, or chronic physical illnesses.

However, in many cases those are just symptoms. The sickness is somewhere else. Maybe one person is sick and poisoning the whole family. Perhaps multiple people are sick, or the family structure itself could be unhealthy even though no specific person is sick.

When I was growing up, I was taught that chronic pain, addiction, and mental illness were individual problems, and that the suffering individual needed to be treated. I was taught that anger, social anxiety, and acting out were individual deficiencies, and that the individual displaying those behaviors needed to be addressed. But as I worked with more and more families and organizations, I began to wonder. What if those problems and behaviors are sometimes symptoms of family sickness? What if diagnosing and treating the individual allows the family sickness to grow, unchecked and untreated? What if focusing on the individual worsens the actual family sickness?

Let me tell you about a young woman I met through my ministry. Let's call her Kayla. The specifics of this story are Kayla's, but I've seen similar narratives play out with a dozen or so young adults.

Kayla is living at home, going to community college, getting pretty good grades, and involved in lots of activities. On the surface, everything seems fine. But it turns out Kayla suffers from severe anxiety and chronic stomachaches that seemingly come out of nowhere. She tries all sorts of diets to deal with the stomachaches, but nothing helps. She also tries the woo-woo stuff, of course. It feels better for a while, but the good feelings never last.

As I get to know Kayla, I ask about how things are going in her immediate family. At first, she just talks about how she admires her father and always listens to his perspective. But after a while, she tells me that her mother often hits her father during arguments. She admits that her father seems to have a problem with women in general, and he often gives Kayla the silent treatment for weeks at a time after she makes minor mistakes. She tells me her parents fight constantly and that her father says he wishes he had never married her mother.

OK. In this case, all the diagnoses in the world, the best possible diet, and a billion aromatherapy sessions will not help this young woman's stomachaches. The anxiety and the chronic pain are just symptoms. Kayla's family is sick.

And of course, her parents are dead set against Kayla moving out. I believe I know why. Kayla's parents don't want her to leave, because with her gone, they'll have to face each other. They'll have to deal with their marital relationship without using their daughter as a bargaining chip or an emotional punching bag. They are afraid (and maybe they should be) of what will happen without her there.

But the family sickness will never heal until Kayla leaves it behind.

So finally, she moves out. I help her do so to the extent I'm able. Kayla remains in contact with her parents but refuses to let them use her as a pawn in their fights. Telling her parents she's moving out is one of the hardest things she's ever had to do. She is shamed, not just by her parents but by her extended family as well. But she moves out anyway. She moves into a space where the family (here "family" refers to the emotionally connected group sharing the house) is relatively healthy. Or at least the family is not abusive.

Within one week, Kayla's anxiety disappears. The stomach-aches are gone in less than a month. These were just symptoms.

Not only that but her parent's relationship begins to heal as they decide to act decently toward each other when Kayla visits. Her parents have lost something, and that loss causes them to consider that perhaps they need to examine their own behavior instead of blaming each other (or Kayla). Now when Kayla visits her parents, family gatherings are enjoyable. She looks forward to seeing the same people she used to approach with dread.

I would say several things happened here. First, Kayla removed herself from a sick family and joined a healthier one. That eliminated her anxiety and stomachaches, which were mere symptoms. Second, when Kayla left, her parents had to deal with the real family sickness. They had to stop fighting over Kayla and face each other. Third, neither of Kayla's parents are bad people. But the family was sick because the parents' relationship had become abusive.

Now I should admit that not all stories have such positive endings. Many times, the family does not heal. Sometimes, instead of doing the hard work of healing, the family just kind of looks for a replacement for the young adult who left. And sometimes symptoms do not disappear so quickly. Symptoms, unfortunately, can linger for quite a while. However, in every single case I've seen, the young person's symptoms declined sharply soon after they were no longer enmeshed in their family's dysfunction.

This is why it's so important to distinguish between sickness and symptoms. If I had thought that Kayla was the one with the problem or if I had tried to diagnose or label her, nothing would have gotten better. She probably would not have improved, and there would have been no opportunity for the family to heal.

Before going any further I need to define what family sickness is: *Sickness is trying to control someone's relationship to someone else.*

A sick family is one in which its members try to control relationships they are not directly involved in. Extreme examples include abusive relationships and oppressive organizations. Mild examples include a grandmother trying to control who her grandchildren marry, a daughter trying to control her parents' fighting, or a boss trying to control two employees' interactions with each other.

Trying to control someone else's relationship with any idea, problem, addiction, issue, value, or goal is also sickness. Using the example from the introduction to this book, if I try to control my friend's drinking, that's sickness. (Yes, even if he is an alcoholic.) If I try to control my business partner's relationship with our business goals, that's also sickness. Even a mother trying to control her daughter's grades is an example.

Now, some forms of family sickness are obviously more severe than others, just like stage-4 cancer is more severe than the common cold. Most of my examples above are more like a cold. Regardless of severity, the problem develops from the attempt to control. It does not develop from simply desiring a positive outcome for someone, and it certainly does not develop from conflict, which is nothing more than two people holding incompatible desires.

So when I want my business partner to succeed, that's healthy. A mother's desire for her daughter to do well in school is healthy, as is a grandmother's wish to see her grandchildren happily married. I want to see my friends released from their addictions, and that's healthy too.

The issue is the attempt to control, but what's surprising is that there might not be one controlling individual. Sometimes a family is sick because there is a "bad guy," a villain who makes the family toxic. But sometimes a family is just sick despite the fact that there is no "bad guy" at all.

When the Family Is Sick Even Though No Individual Family Member Is Sick

Let me tell you a story of a family that was quite sick despite the fact that no single individual in the family was sick. This is a story about the first church where I ever preached, the church my father started. After my father's retirement, they had called a new pastor. He seemed perfectly suited for the job. But for some reason, things never clicked. Eventually, the church got tired of this pastor and asked him to leave.

After that, a rotating cast of four pastors took turns leading the service. Mostly these were retired pastors or pastors in training. In fact, my father had become one of the alternate pastors. This system had been in place for quite some time when I returned to the church. After my father passed away, the church asked me to take his place in the rotating cast. I was happy to do so.

For about a year, everything seemed to be going beautifully. The church started growing again! This was incredible because it had seemed stuck in place for so long. The church recruited a new pastor who was popular and who had served twenty-five years in prison. This guy had one heck of a story about how he had come to God and how God had carried him through his incarceration. He was an excellent fit because our congregation was focused on prison ministry and serving ex-convicts. I was so excited. I felt like I was floating when I walked.

And then, suddenly, it felt like it was all falling apart. I couldn't figure out what was going on. Anxiety was through the roof. Members seemed angry for no reason and were acting out in weird ways. Within one month of hearing the first whispers of trouble—a few complaints here and there about this new pastor—some members of the congregation demanded he be removed from the rotation.

That came out of nowhere. I wondered what had happened. Before I could figure out what was going on, the new pastor announced he would preach his last sermon at the church that coming Sunday. He said he wanted to keep the peace. After the service, we had a meeting of the church council. At that meeting, precisely half the group announced they were quitting. They were upset because they felt the pastor they liked was forced out by the other half of the council. One outgoing member was the guy who held the keys to the building where we worshiped. He set the keys on the table.

Someone from the remaining half said, "Well, Lauren, I guess those keys are yours now. You better pick 'em up." And that's how I became a pastor. The rotation ended and it was just me until our congregation happily merged with the church whose building we shared. The group that split also merged with a neighboring church and still seems to be doing quite well.

So I guess it all worked out, but what had happened? How did our church, which had been stuck for so long, go into such a drastic death spiral right when things seemed to be going well? It looked like we were finally turning the corner, and then bam, it was over. We split in half, right down the middle.

Well, when I talked to the members of the council after the split, I learned quite a lot. I learned there had been two factions in the church for as long as anyone could remember. Everyone kind of knew who these factions and their leaders were, but no one said it out loud. And these factions had been in deep disagreement for years and years.

I asked the man whom I trusted more than anyone else, "How long has the conflict between the leaders of these two groups been going on?" He couldn't remember. I asked, "Since even before my father's retirement?" Definitely, yes. "And what was the conflict about? Do you remember?" No, he couldn't remember what the real issues were or if there even were any real issues.

I had been attending the church council meetings for some time and never knew there was such a deep conflict. Issues were not discussed unless they were so mundane that the eventual vote would be unanimous. If something was controversial, it just got tabled. People never addressed their deep disagreements face to face. They gossiped in their separate factions and tried to figure out how to control the church. On top of that, everyone was hoping I'd stay because my father had started the church, so they presented a cheery facade while I was there.

See, my father was charismatic, so as long as he was there, the two factions of the church didn't compete with each other in the same way. He was the leader, and everyone knew that. But after my father left, the church family struggled to stay well.

I never saw evidence that any individual members involved were sick, certainly not sick enough to break apart an entire church. No, the history and culture of the church were unhealthy. That's why the church couldn't grow. And when it started to grow with this new pastor and me, crisis after crisis seemed to erupt. But there was no real crisis. There was no real issue. The members just realized they'd be happier apart than together.

Other local pastors mentioned to me that, unlike with most church splits, they had heard no gossip. No one outside of our church heard any slander or accusations. I believe that if any individual had been toxic, accusations would have been made. And to be clear, the toxic person would probably be the one making them. But no one accused anyone of anything. No one gossiped. There was not a hint of slander. The church just split cleanly, and then everyone was happier. That was that.

I have never seen a clearer example of a sick family in which there was no bad guy, no villain, no sick individual. The family was just stuck.

In this case, it's possible to come up with a pretty good hypothesis for the original cause of the family sickness. However, I don't think that's important. What's important is to see a sick family for what it is and not waste time trying to identify a villain. There might not be a bad guy. And even if there is a bad guy but you don't deal with the family sickness first, you may identify the wrong person.

When One Person Is Sick and the Whole Family Suffers

In order to explain this dynamic, let me use the most disturbing example—a father who is sexually abusing his children. I present this extreme example because it illustrates truths that are impossible to ignore about sick families. Here is one such truth:

The sexually abusive father often won't show symptoms unless somebody starts to heal. Until then, he will seem to have it all together.

The victims will show some symptoms, obviously. But the most severe symptoms will be shown by those in the family who take emotional responsibility for their father's actions, whether they are victims or not. Those trying to protect the father or the family's reputation (even if only on an internal level) will display the most visible symptoms, which they may transmit to their loved ones.

The reprinted material below details a common example of how that often plays out. This anonymous account comes from an internet forum that hosts online discussions about sexual assault. I have reprinted it because the experience is so typical, and also because it is easier than describing a family I personally know.

I have sat in a room many times with the three grown daughters of a pedophile who sexually abused them as children for years, knowing something was wrong but not what it was. They had a silent agreement to let the grandfather pedophile handle the grandkids, but never to be left alone for a second. Watching him like hawks, to keep his hands off their private parts. All of them had me fooled. Nobody was letting me in on the little secret.

When the eldest daughter, home from college, mustered up the courage to confront him, she gave him an ultimatum: stop abusing the youngest daughter who is your current victim or we go to the sheriff. So he stopped. But he started coaching little girls' tee ball, soccer, and doing church groups. The daughters acknowledge feeling guilty about that, but not enough to tell the people in charge of these groups that this guy was a decade-plus serial rapist of his own children.

What these examples prove is that even the victims themselves cover up for them. The five family members all loved their father. They did not want to see him go to prison. So they essentially said, "We'll protect ourselves from now on but close our eyes to what you do elsewhere."

Whenever I was with this family, I always felt there was something going on. The father spoke nonstop about inane stuff—seemed like you could never get a word in edgewise, but it was with such a soft tone as if it were a gentle breeze when in fact it was this gigantic, awful cancer. It was his control-freaky way of concealing this eight-hundred-pound gorilla in the room. If someone had just said "You raped your daughters for over ten years," that would have finally shut him up. But nobody said a word!

My ex-wife described the terror she felt whenever his favorite TV show came on—a western. Because at the end of that show was when it happened in her bedroom. You have a mother who walked in on him with his fingers up inside her while sitting on his lap in the kitchen. She turned around and walked back out. You're all alone, kid. Nobody's going to help. That's how my ex-wife felt at the end of the show. What are all the other family members thinking as this show is ending and the father goes into her bedroom? She never says to them, "Goodnight, everyone. Daddy's going to sexually assault me now"...

If an investigation had happened because of an accusation at the church or the sports programs, they would have lied for him. Because I did call the sheriff when I discovered all this, so they started an investigation. I got calls from family members, the most menacing from her brother. He left for the Peace Corps for two years after high school. A Catholic mission in some African country. So he didn't have to watch it happening to his little sister. She begged him not to go. She didn't have to say why—it's even worse when nobody's around. So he's lying to the sheriff's office and then angrily calling me to vent. If you are lying to investigators, then you are committing crimes. I don't hate these five enablers, but it proved to be the rift between us that ended everything.

In this example, as so often happens, the man who is sick, the father, shows no symptoms. Well, he seems a little bit "control-freaky." His victims, of course, show some symptoms. But who shows the most serious symptoms? Who goes to the extreme lengths of lying to prosecutors and threatening the one who tells the truth?

Not the victims.

It's the brother, the one who was closest to the youngest daughter. He takes the most emotional responsibility for protecting the family secret. He's the one who acts out the most and who flees to a foreign country. In terms of visible signs of a sick family, he's the one an outside observer would notice first. Yet he is neither the perpetrator nor the victim.

I start off with such a disturbing story because extreme examples show truths in ways that are hard to escape or excuse. Notice what happens when a basically good person, the storyteller who posted this online, tries to solve the problem of a sick family by going after the sick individual at the top. It doesn't work. It doesn't deal with the family sickness, so the family still protects the predator.

The family sickness is trying to control other people's relationships to one another, or other people's relationships to their own values, ideas, or problems. Everything else—the rage, the anxiety, the chronic physical illnesses—these are all just symptoms. The father in this family does everything he can to control everyone's relationships to everyone else, from the way he orchestrates family conversations right down to his implied threat that anyone who speaks up will be responsible for his going to prison.

Will the father ever show symptoms? Oh, he will if any of his victims ever tells the truth, starts to heal, or sets clear boundaries. Once that happens, the father will become offended, perhaps enraged. But he will show symptoms only if the family starts to heal. And then how will the family respond? If the family is like many sick families, they will try to soothe his anger. This, of course, means shutting up the victims.

This is why it's so critical to distinguish between symptoms and sickness. Never assume the one showing symptoms is the one who is sick. I made this mistake over and over again when I started out as a pastor. I thought the person showing the worst symptoms must be either the villain or the victim, and it wasn't true.

Also, if you are the one showing symptoms, don't ever believe that proves you are the one who is sick! Your symptoms are just symptoms. If your family is sick, you will show symptoms even if you are not sick, and even if you are not a victim.

The family in which one sick individual harms the entire group is the easiest example to explain because the distinction between sickness and symptom is so obvious. But in my experience, this type of family is also the least common. In fact, I've known only a few families with just one sick individual. And in those families, the one sick individual held all the economic and social power. Much more common is a family in which its two leaders are sick and in constant conflict.

When the Two Leaders Are Sick and the Rest of the Family Suffers

Here's a common example. The father and mother are emotionally abusive toward each other. The children watch. So instead of one predator, there are two abusers. In such a family, the children often show more severe symptoms than the parents.

The parents may show symptoms of, say, depression or alcoholism. The children, though, may suffer from pathological depression, rage, eating disorders, extreme drug abuse, sexual acting out, or bizarre, chronic physical illnesses. The severity of the symptoms depends on the extent to which the children feel responsible for their parents' behavior.

When I started working with families and dealing with abusive relationships, I heard this often from experienced therapists and pastors: "Children suffer more from watching their parents abuse each other than they do from being abused themselves." And I just didn't believe it. I thought, "This has to be false!" It seemed absurd to me. But as I became more experienced, I realized that it is true.

Steven Stosny, an expert in relationship behaviors, reports he has worked with more than six thousand children from abusive families. Half of those children suffered from anxiety or depression so severe that it interfered with their normal functioning. And they were just as likely to experience anxiety and depression as they would have been if the abuse had never been directed toward them. When the children watch the parents abuse each other, the children suffer.

As I gained even more experience, I realized this problem is not limited to children, nor is it confined to blood relationships. The same thing happens in companies, churches, and even friend groups.

In any emotionally connected group in which the leaders are abusive to each other, the other family members will eventually show symptoms. The most common are various forms of anxiety and depression, and chronic physical ailments such as stomachaches, headaches, and excessive fatigue.

And again, when I started as a pastor, I did not understand this dynamic at all. I thought that if children showed symptoms of being in a sick family, then the parents must be harming the children. Not necessarily so! Quite often, the children are witnesses to their parents harming each other.

When the Family Structure Is Sick

In my experience, most sick families do not have villains at all. I constantly come across families in which no one is abusive, but the family structure is sick. Such a family structure is characterized by incessant conflict, poorly maintained boundaries, communication breakdowns, and a lot of people doing things they hate doing. This is distressingly common in organizations like churches, nonprofits, and businesses that lack healthy competition. These toxic families are marked by total "stuckness." The family seems incapable of moving forward, and everyone feels anxious, frustrated, or burned out.

What the heck is going on? Why is there incessant conflict, even if no individual is sick?

In simple terms, bonding is what's going on. Once people bond, it is as if the relationships have a life of their own, complete with a survival instinct. Relationships strive to maintain themselves. In a healthy family, the resilience of relationship patterns is wonderful. But in an unhealthy family, that same resilience can become harmful. Even if the family is killing all the members with chronic physical and mental illness, the family may resist change.

A family might be sick because of its inherent structure, history, or culture. Often such a family has been sick for as long as anyone can remember, and new blood doesn't change much of anything. As individual family members come and go, the problematic roles they play stay the same. So former family members get replaced by new people who perpetuate the illness, often without realizing it.

If a family has been sick for long enough, the sickness starts to seem normal. The members are so used to it that it may have become invisible. So now let's look at how to identify a sick family.

Signs of a Sick Family

Outlined below are signs that a family is sick. In every case, the signs can show up even if no single individual is sick. These signs provide evidence that is more direct than are some symptoms. After all, a stomachache might be caused by the flu, and rage can be kindled by a bad drug trip. So symptoms might be caused by family sickness, or they might be caused by something more biological or chemical. However, when you see any of these seventeen signs, you are witnessing a sick family.

1. Walking on eggshells.
2. Secrets.
3. Incessant competition for position in the family tree.
4. Criticism, condemnation, and blame.
5. Sarcasm used as a weapon.
6. Labeling people, especially with non-professional diagnoses like "narcissist" or "sociopath."
7. Interventions for the labeled family member.
8. Us-versus-them gossip.
9. Delivering messages for people instead of directly communicating.
10. Constantly trying to save face for those at the top.

11. People showing remorse but not compassion when they hurt others.

12. Accusations of selfishness, laziness, stubbornness, irrationality, and ignorance.

13. Ignoring consent. Trying to make decisions for people without their input and using people as chess pieces in conflicts.

14. Constant unsolicited advice.

15. No humor or playfulness. Everything is always "serious."

16. Not defining oneself. When someone states a position or identity, others do not respond by stating their own position. Instead, they focus on attacking or belittling.

17. Conflicts seem locked in place. No matter what the conflict was originally about or where it started, it usually ends up involving the same antagonists playing the same roles.

One: Walking on Eggshells

Gut feelings are not always right, but this is the one gut feeling no one should ever ignore. When you feel like you are walking on eggshells around someone, especially if you feel it from an entire group, you are dealing with a sick family. In fact, you may very well be dealing with outright abuse.

When I interview abuse victims, I always ask one question that gets to the heart of the matter: "Do you ever feel like you are walking on eggshells?" Based on the answer to that question, I find out a lot about what's going on in the family.

Why is this feeling of walking on eggshells so important? Your intuition may not always be accurate, but it is always accurate about *you*. Any warnings your intuition gives you about yourself are true. Now, that doesn't mean your gut feelings about other people are necessarily the truth, but they are valid pointers toward how you are thinking and behaving.

So what does it mean when you feel you are walking on eggshells? What is your intuition telling you? Your intuition is telling you that you are censoring yourself. You may even be shaming yourself. You are trying to make yourself small and unthreatening so a predator does not notice you. This would be fine if you were in a room with a silverback gorilla. It is not fine when you are with a group of people you care about.

If you are walking on eggshells, then either other people are trying to control you, or you are trying to control other people. There is no in-between.

Now, as you read this, you might think, *But if I stop walking on eggshells and say how I really feel, there will be an explosion. There will be a crisis, and I don't want that.* That's an important point, and saying the "wrong" thing could get you stonewalled or scapegoated.

But the hard truth about those explosions and crises is this: In a sick family, explosions happen whenever anything changes, including changes for the better. So if a crisis develops, it's not clear whether the family is getting better or worse, or if it's just part of a repetitive up-and-down pattern. And this is the key to how families stay sick. They resist change at all costs. The family doesn't explode because something bad happened. The family explodes because the familiar dynamic is changing.

A healthy family doesn't need to resist change, because it can adapt. In a healthy family, you do not feel like you are walking on eggshells. You feel like the floor is solid beneath you and that the steps you take have purpose. For those accustomed to walking on eggshells, this feeling of solidity might seem almost boring at first. This is because the usual pattern is that, for a while, you feel like you are floating on air. Then an argument happens or someone says "no." And suddenly, the very earth beneath your feet feels fragile. That can be an exciting roller coaster ride, but it's also unhealthy.

Boring isn't the worst thing in the world. You always need firm ground you can return to. In healthy families, everyone feels grounded. And from that position of security and strength, people can learn to soar without worrying that the rest of the group might clip their wings.

Two: Secrets

Many years ago, a close friend of mine became addicted to cocaine. In his well-off family, keeping up appearances was important. So for years he didn't discuss his habit. He had gotten addicted in a far-off big city, and when he returned home, many of his closest friends didn't know about his struggle. Of course, he wasn't supposed to tell them, and neither was anyone else. His friends, then, would ask him if he wanted to go out and party. He would just sit there and suffer, trying to make up some excuse as to why he couldn't participate. He censored himself, hid his inner turmoil, and stacked dishonesty upon dishonesty.

I don't know if my friend's addiction recovery was all that painful, but the shame of having to cover it up certainly was. Secrets are always connected to shame.

This is a good time to point out that when I discuss the signs of a sick family, I am not yet offering up solutions. Solutions will be presented in later chapters. It's tempting to think the solution here is to reveal the family secrets—to just put them all out in the open. That might help or it might hurt, but it doesn't address the problem.

Sure, secrets in and of themselves do cause certain problems. For instance, secrets divide the family between those in the know and those in the dark. Secrets also destroy people's ability to be open and spontaneous. It's no fun at all to always have to remember what you can talk about and what you can't.

The deeper problem with secrets is that the family regards some things as so shameful that they can't be spoken aloud, which is ridiculous. Let's say the secret is some action or habit that caused harm. How is refusing to discuss the harm helping anyone? How does either the victim or the aggressor move on if they can't even acknowledge what happened? And if the secret doesn't involve harm, then what could possibly be so bad that it can't even be mentioned?

The level of shame that requires a secret to be held can exist only in a family in which people are straining to control relationships that are none of their business. And the ultimate examples of a relationship that is none of my business are "what people will say," "what the neighbors think," or "what everyone will gossip about." If I am so sick that I am trying to control what strangers believe, then my sickness is not going to be healed by a mere confrontation or a rebellious act like airing out the family's dirty laundry.

Blowing open the family's secrets may lead to some healing, or it may just lead to a big mess. Remember I'm not talking about solutions yet—we'll get there in the next couple of chapters. For now, I'm just pointing out the signs of a healthy family versus the signs of an unhealthy one.

A healthy family doesn't require you to keep track of what you can and can't say, doesn't ask you to remember every little comment you've ever made, and doesn't expect you to constantly censor yourself. There is no need for secrets in a healthy family because nothing is seen as so shameful that it can't be discussed. Secrets are perhaps the most obvious sign of a shame-ridden family, a clear red flag that a group, organization, or relationship is sick.

Three: Incessant Competition

Competition is fine, but constant warfare is a clear warning sign of family sickness. In most sick families I've encountered, there was a distressingly high level of conflict for position or dominance. This excessive competition happens between both men and women, although the competitions typically play out differently among the different genders.

The big problem with battles over status is that they never seem to resolve into simple, one-on-one confrontations. It's never like a Western film in which the two men go outside of the saloon and have a gunfight. Instead, the family battle is fought socially. Both competitors try to line up allies and subordinates, tending to use manipulation, coercion, or outright slander as their primary weapons. Family members who don't want to get involved end up stuck in the middle of a war they have neither the desire nor the fortitude to fight. Everyone gets stressed out and anxious.

A lot of people seem to believe everyone wants to be in charge—that everyone secretly wants to be at the top of the family pyramid. But I doubt that very much. Most people seem to find a preferred role, which often relates to the sibling role they played in their blood family. And they are often pretty happy if they stay in that role.

This observation may be true even of many primates. Biology professor and researcher Robert Sapolsky set out to answer a question about social hierarchies in animal species. He wondered, *Who is more stressed? The dominant animals in a group, or the low-ranking animals?* Interestingly, he found that, well, it depends. In many cases, what mattered was not where in the dominance hierarchy an animal was situated. What mattered was how stable the hierarchy was. Many animals, not just people, are happier with stability than being on top.

In a healthy family, there is some stability to roles, and people are genuinely happy in the role they play. Also, people get positive reinforcement for playing their roles well. In healthy social circles, organizations, and relationships, every role matters. This is probably the primary reason you don't see excessive competition for status in high-functioning groups. When you are secure in your role, know that your role matters, and are confident you can play it well, you are much less susceptible to envy or jealousy.

Four: Criticism, Condemnation, and Blame

Dale Carnegie had a famous motto: "Avoid the three Cs. Do not criticize, condemn, or complain."

Relationship expert Steven Stosny often points out that the abuser's motto is, "I feel bad and it's your fault."

Carnegie also said, "Any fool can criticize, condemn, and complain—and most fools do. But it takes character and self-control to be understanding and forgiving."

Similarly, Stosny asserts that anyone can acquire an abusive mindset. All that's required is to avoid taking responsibility and instead habitually blame others.

Can a family be abusive without a clear abuser? Yes, and it happens in the same way an individual becomes abusive. All that needs to happen is for repeated situations to develop in which people avoid responsibility and spread blame. The whole family can get caught up in a game of criticism and condemnation that no one wants to play.

There is a difference between assigning fault and taking responsibility. To take responsibility simply means that you accept that you have the power to respond. Criticism, condemnation, and blame, on the other hand, are all versions of pointing the finger at someone and saying, "It's your fault." And yes, you can blame yourself, too. Self-blame isn't helpful either because it lets everyone else avoid responsibility.

Say I wake up one morning and find a baby on my doorstep. Is it my fault this baby is on my doorstep? Clearly not. Is this baby on my doorstep my responsibility? *Hmm.* That's a more challenging question. The answer is not so obvious. But that's OK because this question is meant to show the difference between fault and responsibility.

Let's go back to the definition of responsibility. To take responsibility means to accept that you have the power to respond. Do I have the power to respond to this baby left on my doorstep? The answer is yes. It's not my fault, but it is my responsibility.

In unhealthy families, people avoid responsibility and instead spend their time figuring out who or what to blame. These are the phrases you'll hear: "Who is at fault?" "Why do we always get the short end of the stick?" "Why do things always go wrong?" "Who told you to do this?" "Why are you always doing that?" "Why don't you ever...?" But despite all the criticism, condemnation, and blame, no one accepts that they have the power to respond.

In a healthy family, people don't blame but instead take responsibility, so there is no need to criticize, condemn, or complain. In healthy families, when things go wrong—even when people *do* wrong—individuals figure out how they can do better. In healthy families, conflict, disappointment, and failure often lead to creativity, which is good since conflict, failure, and disappointment are inevitable. Those setbacks can produce new ideas about how to solve problems and stay connected.

Five: Sarcasm

Wait, isn't a sense of humor a good thing? Yes, it is. And sometimes, sarcastic humor is just playful and clever.

But most of the time, sarcasm is about managing appearances. It's about trying to come off as smarter, wittier, and less vulnerable than others. Sarcasm is usually evidence of distance, evidence of a family whose members seek acceptable ways to communicate hostility or frustration. And the hostility always gets communicated, as does the additional message that somehow the recipient of that hostility shouldn't respond to it for what it is.

Everyone pretends it's just a joke. But often the joker is frustrated, not so much that they aren't getting their way but that they aren't even being heard or noticed. Or perhaps the joker is trying to jockey for position in a way that won't be seen as naked ambition. In the worst cases, sarcasm is used to undermine someone else. And if that someone is accused of being too sensitive after claiming the humor stings, then the family is certainly sick.

Sarcasm in and of itself is not a red flag. But humor that's meant to sting is a red flag, and such humor usually surfaces as sarcasm. But don't assume the person using sarcasm is the one with the problem. It's rarely that simple. Often the sarcastic one has defaulted to that method because they feel they can't get attention any other way. Or the family is just too unstable, so everyone feels uncomfortable bringing out their genuine grievances. They react by delivering veiled jabs in the form of jokes that are about 90 percent truth and 10 percent humor.

In a healthy family, humor doesn't sting. Humor is just playful and funny, like pandas wrestling in popular online videos. And yes, in a healthy family, humor is also common.

Six: Labeling

Along with walking on eggshells, labeling is one of the signs that a family is so unhealthy that it might be outright abusive. But the person who is being labeled is usually not the problem. The person getting labeled is more likely the scapegoat.

Consider this example. No psychiatrist would accept their spouse as a patient. It would be impossible for the psychiatrist to be objective. And yet many people label their spouses and their ex-spouses with various kinds of psychological diagnoses: narcissism, borderline, codependence, anxiety disorder, and so on. It's kind of funny to go on relationship internet forums where pages and pages of respondents complain about "my narcissist." Strangely, none of those complaining ever seem to label themselves "codependent" or "borderline."

The problem of labeling has become commonplace in American culture. I can't even imagine anymore what politics would sound like without all the misleading labels: racist, socialist, elitist, communist. Labeling is so common that I worry people are starting to perceive it as normal.

Labeling is not normal, and it is not healthy. And labeling becomes outright dangerous when the labels are black and white with no shades of gray in between. You are either the scapegoat or the golden child, the empath or the narcissist, the selfish jerk or the selfless martyr. Others define you by your supposed intentions, which of course you can never disprove. In the sickest families, not only are people labeled as if they are all bad or all good, but the labels constantly switch. One day a kid is the golden child, and the next day they are considered the epitome of evil.

In a healthy family, no one is ever seen to be all bad or all good. People are understood to be a complex mix. In a healthy family, intentions and motivations are rarely discussed. Instead, the family focuses on actions and consequences, habits, and long-term results. When failures, problems, and conflicts occur, a healthy family does not immediately try to label someone as the villain. That energy is better spent figuring out how to change the environment, so the problems do not reoccur.

Seven: Interventions

Interventions almost never work. They often provoke the opposite of the desired results because they cause the subject to feel like a child and then to act like one. The most common response to an intervention is passive-aggressive rebellion.

Every intervention I've ever heard of backfired. A bunch of my friends tried an intervention with an alcoholic who was part of our group. As a result, he drank more and got even angrier when drunk. A family I know was struggling with an elderly relative. They tried to intervene to get her to seek medical care more often. Instead, she moved hundreds of miles away so they could no longer check up on her. A close friend's mother was driving away her adult children because of her resentment and controlling behavior. The siblings tried an intervention. Afterward, the mother became so vicious that most of the siblings cut off contact with her altogether.

Some interventions somewhere must have worked. Otherwise, no one would participate in them. But even if, by some miracle, an intervention is successful, it is a clear and obvious signal that the family is sick. The mere existence of an intervention means some members of the group are trying to control other people's relationships to one another.

In healthy families, people lead by example. I would argue that leadership by example is the only real form of leadership. In a healthy family, those perceived as leaders stay connected to everyone else while clearly defining their own boundaries. Someone who is suffering and deemed to be in need of intervention is more likely to change their behavior in a thriving environment where they see constant examples of good behavior.

Eight: Us-versus-Them Gossip

Every family gossips. In a healthy family, gossip is mere entertainment and serves to bind people together. In an unhealthy family, gossip is used to line up allies against the opposing side. Such gossip usually focuses on people's intentions, motivations, and character, because there is no way to bring up actual evidence of intentions, motivations, and character. So it's possible to create a caricature of a person that turns into something close to an outright fabrication.

Examples include social media chat groups where participants talk about someone who isn't in the chat, or meetings in which the person being discussed isn't invited. These discussions rarely involve facts or even actions the person took. Instead, they often entail unrelated incidents, vague insinuations, and lengthy complaints about comments taken out of context.

My experience may not be universal, but us-versus-them gossip was the first red flag I saw at every unhealthy business, sick nonprofit organization, or dysfunctional government agency I've worked with or visited. There shouldn't be opposing sides in an organization that is supposed to have a clear mission and goals. And if there are sides, they shouldn't be the first thing I notice when I come to visit or discuss a project.

It certainly shouldn't be easier for people to talk to *me* about their conflicts than to one another! Us-versus-them gossip pervades bureaucratic families such as nonprofits and government agencies. And I believe such gossip is hard on the idealistic folks who often seek such jobs because it is the antithesis of what they thought they signed up for.

Healthy nonprofits do exist, and functioning bureaucracies are real. In a healthy family, whether at the workplace or at home, people communicate directly, and conflicts are discussed openly. Us-versus-them gossip is rare in healthy groups because conflicts move around the family instead of becoming frozen in place. If your family is healthy, you will find yourself on different teams and different sides depending on the issue. As a result, most of the gossip will just be entertaining.

Nine: Delivering Messages

This one is a surprise to a lot of folks, since many grew up in families in which it was normal to deliver messages. "Go tell your sister..." "Go ask your auntie..." And if the message is just about sitting down to dinner, then that isn't a problem. But when the messages are more complex, and especially if the family is an organization, business, church, or collective, being asked to deliver messages is a bright-red flag.

The first problem with delivering a message for someone is that its meaning gets lost. Context and subtlety are eliminated or, in some cases, twisted. The messenger always changes the message a little bit, and often to suit their own needs and desires.

So what's going on? Why would anyone ask someone else to communicate for them? The issue is that the asker is avoiding confrontation. In a worst-case scenario, if you are asked to deliver a message, it's because the asker wants you to take the heat for the recipient's reaction. In a best-case scenario, the one asking is oblivious to the consequences of encouraging people to play the telephone game instead of communicating directly.

In large organizations, of course, tasks get delegated. A manager might get a directive and be asked to figure out the details. But in a healthy organization, that still does not devolve into a situation in which the manager is expected to do the higher-up's communication for them. It should be clear who is responsible for what. Maybe those at the top set the goals and the general tone, and yes, the managers figure out the details. But it is still the leaders' responsibility to articulate their vision.

In a sick organization, again, it's not that delivering messages for people is a huge problem in and of itself. The problem is that some people are so afraid of confrontation and what such confrontation might lead to that they are unwilling to speak and listen. That's where the sickness lies.

Confrontation is inevitable because conflict is inevitable. However, confrontation by itself rarely leads to a solution. It's what happens after and around the confrontation that matters. Still, in a healthy family, people are expected to face their fears of confrontation, and everyone understands that confrontations can be painful. But we all need to learn to tolerate that pain, just like we tolerate the pain of exercise and brushing our teeth.

Ten: Saving Face

In my experience, every church, artistic collective, and business in which creative frustration was rampant featured a "peacemonger" for a leader. A peacemonger is someone who always tries to smooth things over, who tries to hold the family together at all costs, whose primary concern is making sure no feathers get ruffled, who always wants to default to consensus decision-making instead of confronting hard issues, and whose highest value seems to be saving face.

But conflict exists whether it is stated out loud or not. It exists whether or not people admit it. Conflict happens anytime one person wants one thing, and another person wants something else. And in the end, trying too hard to smooth things over worsens conflicts because the only way to keep everyone happy is to turn what should be a conflict between two people into a conflict that involves the whole group.

If someone is unhappy and I, as the leader, want to smooth over their unhappiness without letting them confront the issue or the person themselves, I don't have any good options. I can enlist the aid of other members in the group to calm the person down. I can attempt to make people like each other. I can ignore divisions in the hope that the conflicts will just go away. I can try to make everyone get along without ever letting everyone say how they actually feel. The end result of all this manipulation and misdirection is that almost every member of the group ends up being involved in the conflict, so now the conflict is too complex to resolve.

When conflict occurs in healthy families, the goal is to reduce the number of people involved. So an emphasis on saving face is never a good sign. In a sick family, saving face for those at the top is more important than progress toward goals or adherence to stated values. A family that prioritizes saving face is telling its members that pretending to be well is more important than being well.

Eleven: Remorse

I'm spending some time on this one because, as a pastor, I've learned that most people do not know the difference between remorse and compassion.

Here is the difference. Let's say I harmed you. Remorse focuses on how bad I feel because of the harm I caused. So remorse devalues me. I devalue myself by focusing on how bad I feel. And when I feel devalued, I am more likely to be harmful or even abusive. Remember that the motto of an abusive mindset is, "I feel bad and it's your fault." So the worse I feel about myself, the more likely I am to be abusive.

Abusive people usually have low self-esteem, although they might present a surface-level narcissistic bravado. They often suffer from anxiety because they are trying to control what cannot be controlled. And they might even believe that anyone with reasonable self-esteem is selfish, because they have a low opinion of their own self.

Now, let's say again that I harmed you. Compassion is focused on how you, the person I hurt, feel. Since I am not focused on myself at all but on you, I do not feel any worse about myself. Compassion focuses on what I can do to repair the hurt and prevent it from happening again. Since taking action to solve a problem causes me to feel better about myself, focusing on my actions improves my self-esteem.

A compassionate person's self-esteem improves even though they focus on other people. Compassionate people have lessening anxiety because they focus on understanding others instead of trying to control them. Compassionate people also have less anxiety because they focus on what they can control—their own actions.

Never forget that a person who devalues themselves is much more likely to become harmful than a person who values themselves. The more someone focuses on how bad they feel for hurting you, the more likely they are to hurt you again.

If you grew up in a sick family, you may have been taught to think that you should show remorse when you've done something wrong. You may have been taught that you should focus on how bad you feel. This is how shame, guilt, and anxiety operate. And it's all misguided.

When you've done something wrong, you should not focus on how you feel at all! Instead, focus on what you need to do to repair the harm. Focus on understanding how the person you hurt feels and thinks. Think about what you will do differently next time. And yes, when someone demands remorse from you instead of compassion, their demands are unhealthy. They just want you to submit.

In a healthy family, people sometimes show remorse, but they always show compassion. When someone violates a boundary or causes harm, they focus on how to repair the harm and make sure it doesn't happen again. In most healthy organizations, this often means evaluating traditions and rules. An emphasis on genuine compassion is an obvious sign that a group is healthy.

Twelve: Accusations

People have an unfortunate habit of believing that if there is an accusation, there must be some truth to it. When an accusation is specific about a concrete action, that might be the case. But accusations such as selfish, lazy, stubborn, and irrational are not concrete. They attempt to describe an individual's character. They are also open to interpretation and impossible to prove or disprove. Any action or inaction can be interpreted as laziness, selfishness, or irrationality if someone is determined to reach those conclusions.

Even in healthy families, people sometimes do the wrong thing. So a healthy family might accuse a person of specific misbehavior. But when someone's character is being assassinated, more often the accuser is guilty and not the accused. It's impossible to fully step into someone else's mindset. Most of the time, people who make unfounded accusations are just projecting. As a result, accusations often say more about the accuser than about anyone else.

The accusations, though, say the most about the family as a whole. Sick families feature endless accusations for the same reason they endure endless criticism and complaints. Family members are focused on controlling others and avoiding responsibility.

Thirteen: Ignoring Consent

If you want to say no, that's a good enough reason to say no. If someone else wants to say no to you, that's a good enough reason for them to say no. That's pretty much the beginning of understanding consent.

This might come as a surprise, but in healthy families, people say no a lot. In the healthiest organizations I've seen, whether for-profit or not-for-profit, people say no around 80 percent of the time.

Warren Buffet said, "The difference between successful people and really successful people is that really successful people say no to almost everything." In any healthy organization that is also growing, people are going to come up with a lot of ideas. To find out what works and what doesn't, folks have to make a lot of asks. That means hearing some version of "no" quite often.

In healthy families, people feel free to ask for what they want or need, and others feel free to say yes or no. That freedom means people get used to hearing the word "no." Of course, if you are in a group that is not trying to expand or change, you may find patterns that everyone is happy with, and you won't have to hear "no" so often. Sometimes friend groups are like this, and it's fine. But most vital organizations seek to advance, evolve, or grow, and that means accepting and welcoming change.

The opposite of a family in which everyone learns to hear the word "no" is one in which people try to make decisions about others without their input. This is a family where some faction that considers itself the enlightened leaders gets together and has long discussions about members who aren't present. They debate what the absent members should do, how they should change, what's wrong with their relationships, and so on.

In the most destructive version of this sick family, people are used as chess pieces in conflicts. When an unhealthy organization reaches that point, you have only two choices: (1) stay, and suffer serious anxiety, rage, or depression, or (2) leave.

Fourteen: Unsolicited Advice

If my car breaks down and someone gives me advice on how to fix it, that is not a sign of an unhealthy relationship. What I'm discussing here is when people tell one another how to think or feel in an attempt to be "helpful." That's worse than unhelpful. It's controlling, and it often goes hand in hand with being a peacemonger.

In a healthy family, people are understood to have their own strengths, goals, and abilities and to know what's in their own best interests. Advice is fine if it is solicited. If you have a goal, and someone is an expert on how to reach that goal, of course it's fine to ask for guidance. Constant unsolicited advice, however, is a red flag, especially if it involves people telling you what your goals or values should be.

Fifteen: No Humor

A clear sign of a healthy family is playfulness. Laughing feels good. Smiling makes you happy. Seeing other people smile and hearing other people laugh lifts everyone's spirits. Laughter is a prehistoric form of communication that shows everyone, "See? There's no danger. It's no big deal."

So everyone enjoys playfulness and knows it's a good sign. This is a great example, though, of why it's not a good idea to try to heal a sick family by forcing the signs to change. If you try to force playfulness, you might just end up with sarcasm. If you try to force people to stop being serious, you'll probably just end up persuading them to avoid responsibility.

In a sick family, there is often an oppressive air of seriousness. When people are serious all the time, they are not trying to merely control each other. They are trying to control the entire environment. It's as if they are trying to manipulate the oxygen in the room. Seriousness indicates a lack of creativity and trust, as well as a silent, hopeless desperation.

Think about every time you've ever watched a parent try to force a kid to be serious. The best-case scenario is that the kid becomes bored. Worst case, the kid goes ballistic. Yes, people need to be serious at certain times and in specific settings. But if a family is always serious minded, then it is probably just stuck in place.

Sixteen: Not Defining Oneself

A great way to gauge the health of your family is to choose any issue that is controversial and simply state your position in a group setting. State it without bringing up the opposing side, without mentioning arguments against it, and without any hint of condescension or passive-aggression. Then watch how people respond.

In a truly healthy family, people will respond by listening. No matter how much they might disagree with you, they will focus on making sure they understood what you said and why you said it.

In a fairly healthy family, people will respond to your self-definition by defining themselves. In other words, if you stake out a position on a controversial issue, people will respond by defining their own position on that issue without necessarily arguing with you. And if they do argue with you, it will be respectful.

In an unhealthy family, people will focus on your statement without defining their own values. They will say things like, "But how can you say that when just last week you said such-and-such?" or "That doesn't make sense because of this," or "That's a really emotional statement," or "You say that because you are a..."

And in an outright abusive family, people will stonewall you, belittle you, or raise their voice at you to drown out your opinion.

Another way of looking at it is to ask yourself this: *Do I feel free to say what I think? Or do I constantly have to worry what side it puts me on to express my opinion?* If you have to worry about what side you're taking, your family is unhealthy. In healthy families, the sides are always changing depending on the conflict or issue.

Seventeen: Conflicts Seem Locked in Place

Every family has occasional conflict. That is unavoidable. In fact, conflict is good because conflict brings the opportunity for growth. And conflict exists even if people never admit that it does.

What might be surprising is that in healthy families, conflict wanders around the family. You can never predict where it's going to break out next or who will be involved. There are different protagonists and antagonists every time. This makes the family flexible and adaptable.

In a family that's stuck, the exact opposite occurs. Whenever a conflict arises in such families, no matter its source and/or content, the same two factions line up on each side of an issue. It doesn't even seem conscious, and it is certainly not rational. People just seem to know what side they're on without having to think about it. Due to the lack of flexibility, the family cannot adapt to new challenges.

The clearest example I know of this type of stuck family was the church I mentioned earlier. After that church split up, I found out how things had been working for years. The church council was made up of twelve people. Every time any controversial issue arose, without exception, six lined up on one side of the issue and six lined up on the other. Meanwhile, they always avoided voting on anything difficult or controversial. Instead they covered up conflicts and voted only on the issues that everyone agreed on.

And of course, the council members also bitterly resisted any attempt to expand the church council. That would have thrown the whole system into chaos.

As I explained before, this church split in half. I believe everyone would have been happier if they had just split a decade sooner. I never found any evidence suggesting that anyone in the church was the villain. The family didn't include any sick individuals, as far as I could tell. No, the family itself was sick. It was stuck, unable to change, unable to move forward, unable to even tolerate an open, honest conversation.

Families in which conflicts are locked in place do often talk a good game about togetherness and inclusivity. "This family stays together no matter what!" But they aren't really together. They are just stuck together. In a healthy family, no one feels stuck. People stay because they want to, not because they can't stand to let their side lose some battle that no one even understands anymore.

Even in an Abusive Relationship, There Might Not Be a Bad Guy

I want to end this chapter by returning once more to the point that even the sickest families might not have a villain.

I rent out most of the rooms in my home, and I often joke that I have discovered the landlord's secret to happiness: never rent to couples.

During an unfortunate five-year stretch, on eight (yes, eight!) separate occasions, the police came to my house to deal with domestic violence. Now when the police receive a domestic violence call, they show up in force, often with a dozen cars. It feels like an invasion, and that's because those calls can be so dangerous for the responders.

If I move beyond domestic violence and consider emotional abuse, by my count, I've now lived with a total of seven different abusive couples.

Here's where things get interesting. All of these abusive relationships have ended. So what happened afterward? Did the "abuser" find a new victim? Did the "victim" just keep bouncing from abusive relationship to abusive relationship? To my slight surprise, the answer to those questions is a resounding no. With the exception of one serial abuser, once these abusive relationships ended, each individual was all right.

Also, throughout most of those relationships, I observed that both partners seemed to take turns playing the roles of victim and abuser. When the relationship ended, both people stopped playing either role.

The individuals were not the problem. Their relationship was the problem.

As a pastor who does prison ministry, I have witnessed so many abusive families. Dealing with domestic violence is a normal part of my job. Very few people continue getting into abusive relationships, repeating the same mistakes over and over. Chronically abusive individuals do exist, but they seem quite rare.

On top of that, I've seen several examples of couples who became abusive, but then they seemed OK after they broke up. They did pretty well until they got back together, thinking they had both dealt with their issues. But as soon as they were reunited, the old relationship patterns showed up with renewed force.

Hopefully, it wasn't a situation as serious as abuse, but I'm sure you've observed similar relationship dynamics. Maybe you've returned to a former relationship or an old family setting that brought back patterns of feeling, thinking, and behaving that you hoped you had left behind. The feelings could even return just by being reminded of the past.

Here's another question worth asking yourself: *How many times have I seen a friend's relationship end and, after a realistic grieving period, the friend seemed better off?* Maybe you knew only one side of the story, so you just figured the partner was the bad guy. But how about a situation in which two of your friends ended a relationship? How often, again, after a reasonable period for grief, did both of your friends seem better off?

If there really was a bad guy, how did both people end up happier post-breakup? When this happens, it seems to me the only reasonable conclusion is that the relationship itself was sick, not the two individuals in it.

This is my plea and my prayer to you. Some people are chronically abusive, but there are far more abusive relationships than there are abusive people. There are personality disorders, but you are much more likely to encounter a toxic family than a toxic person. Whether you are looking in the mirror or thinking about someone else, start by examining family sickness. Please don't ever start by attempting to diagnose the individual.

CHAPTER 2

THE FAMILY'S RESPONSE TO ITS OWN SICKNESS

The family's response to individual symptoms can be even worse than the symptoms themselves. The family member with the most severe or most attention-grabbing symptoms often gets "diagnosed" or labeled, almost becoming a scapegoat. Once an individual's symptoms are diagnosed as a medical problem, a mental health issue, or a personality disorder, the family sickness itself is ignored. So even if a symptom gets "fixed" in one individual, it just pops up somewhere else in the family as a new symptom.

NINE YEARS AFTER MY FATHER DIED, HE VISITED ME IN a dream. Or rather, I visited him. In my dream, I drove to see him at a hotel. He was watching a movie on TV, and we had been eating pizza. I was about to head off to somewhere that seemed important after I had eaten nearly all the pizza.

There was one piece of pepperoni left. I was telling him

that he could eat it if he wanted to, but if he didn't, I would certainly enjoy having it for breakfast in the morning. My father pointed out that half of another pizza was left. At first, I thought the other pizza had just cheese and pineapples, but then I realized it had green peppers too. I explained that green peppers are bad for my stomach, telling him, "So I can't eat this pizza here."

I cannot remember what movie he was watching or where I was off to. But I woke up in the middle of this conversation discombobulated, still believing that I was out at that hotel. My room and house felt unfamiliar. My bed seemed strange. I couldn't figure out where I was for a good minute.

Like I said, my father died nine years ago. When I perform funeral rites in the role I inherited from him, people often ask some version of the question: "How long does the grieving process take?" I always tell them I don't know, but I can now say that, based on my experience, the process could take at least nine years.

This was not the first dream I had about my father since his death, but it is the first that was not either sad or creepy. Two elements stand out when I remember how positive an experience it was. First, we were at a hotel, traveling. My happiest memories of him involve our road trips across the state and the country. Second, here's something that anyone who ever knew my father will recognize—food is involved. He loved to preach about how, in the Gospel of Luke, Jesus is always eating. I sometimes think that if my father hadn't become a pastor, he would have been a chef.

Oh, and the food was my favorite, pizza? Yes, this was a good dream.

I was talking once with a friend about his rock band that had just broken up. They had seemed successful, at least to me. His comment, though, saddened me: "You know, I try my best to remember the good times, but all I can remember are the fights and the arguments." With my father, nine years after his death, it's the opposite. I can't even remember the conflicts anymore. All I can remember are the good times and the positive feelings.

And it's not that my father and I never had conflicts. He was easy to love from a distance, but it was harder up close. The difficulties often revolved around the same two problems—his drinking and his depression. These two issues, though, were symptoms of the family sickness he inherited. When my father was five years old, his father, who was a mafia associate, disappeared. I further describe my father's family of origin in a later chapter, but for now that's enough information for you to imagine the intergenerational trauma he had to overcome.

So yes, I had conflicts with my father. On a purely intellectual level, I remember that our relationship was often difficult. But on an emotional level, I don't feel anything negative. My father's depression and alcohol abuse were quite real, but they were just symptoms. I have no lingering issues with him, not because those symptoms were mild but because the family's response to the symptoms was healthy.

When a family has to deal with a symptom like mental illness or addiction and all the associated behaviors, there are two general ways the family will respond. The family may respond with a combination of shame, revenge, and enabling. On the other hand, the family may respond with openness, clear boundaries, and forgiveness.

Forgiveness versus Enabling and Boundaries versus Revenge

There is a reason I put forgiveness and boundaries on one side and revenge and enabling on the other. Forgiving people and setting boundaries go hand in hand because they both aim to break the cycle of suffering. They are about responsibility, and they are future focused. On the other hand, shame-based responses, such as revenge and enabling, perpetuate the cycle of suffering and focus on the past.

To illustrate this, let me start by talking about forgiveness and about one of the most frustrating things I sometimes hear from churches. Every so often, a church will try to deal with domestic violence by convincing the abuser to apologize. After the apology, the church will then tell the victim that they must now forgive the abuser.

There are several problems here, one of the most important being that this isn't even forgiveness. Forgiveness only follows repentance, and repentance does not mean saying, "I'm sorry." To repent means to turn around, to change directions. If someone has committed acts of domestic violence and their habitual behavior hasn't changed, then any attempt to forgive them isn't forgiveness at all. It's just tolerance.

If someone has changed their behavior and you refuse to accept that reality by continuing to bring up their past, then you perpetuate the cycle of violence, trauma, and suffering. You make it more likely that they will return to their past behaviors. Conversely, if someone has not changed, then trying to "forgive" them just perpetuates the same cycle of violence, trauma, and suffering because you've proven to them that you will tolerate their behavior. In other words, you are enabling.

Abuse is habitual behavior. So repentance involves changing habits, not just saying sorry. When churches demand victims forgive their abusers despite the victims having no real evidence of repentance, those churches are endorsing the exact opposite of forgiveness.

Boundaries and revenge are opposites in the same way that forgiveness and enabling are opposites. Revenge perpetuates the cycle of family sickness in obvious ways, whereas setting good boundaries interrupts that cycle. Openness and shame have a similar dynamic. Shame perpetuates intergenerational trauma by hiding it so it can never be addressed, whereas openness allows healing to be possible.

Labeling the Individual

Here is yet another way that shame, revenge, and enabling are similar. They all rely on labeling an individual as "sick," and acting as though the sick individual is the whole problem. Shame says, "If we could only hide this person..." Revenge says, "If we could only get rid of this person..." Enabling says, "If only this person got the perfect combination of love, support, and firmness, then they would change." Of course, none of those attitudes are realistic because none of them even acknowledge that the family, organization, or relationship has a problem.

So what does any of this have to do with my father's death and the dream in which I visited him?

My father often went to funerals with me. Funerals are a bigger part of a pastor's job than people might realize. We talked about his own funeral, which he knew would happen sooner or later. He told me several times, "Lauren, at my funeral, I don't want a bunch of people getting up there and talking about what a good man I was. Promise me you won't let that happen." I made him that promise, and I kept it.

See, shame is a funny thing. If I had tried to whitewash

my father's story at his own funeral, that would have been a shame-based response. He didn't want that. He wasn't ashamed of his real, complicated, multidimensional story. And he didn't want other people to be ashamed if they had lived similar stories. In fact, that had been a big part of his ministry. The church council's president once told me, "I don't think I've ever met anyone less judgmental than your father."

So at my father's funeral, I told a complex, difficult story instead of hiding anything. I refused to label him an alcoholic just like I refused to label him a good man. I brought up his accomplishments and the reasons he was loved. Yet some people wished I hadn't brought up his drinking, his growing up without a father, his depression, or anything negative. They wanted a simplistic story, one that would let them feel comfortable. But refusal to discuss my father's suffering would imply that his issues were so terrible as to be unmentionable. That is part of why he made me promise there wouldn't be "a bunch of people getting up there and talking about what a good man I was."

This is what's hidden in even the positive labels we often attach to individuals. They hide parts of the story, and they often keep both the individual and the group focused on what's hidden. This is shame's terrible legacy. You can't hide something without having to think about it all the time!

So in the spirit of openness, forgiveness, and solid boundaries, these are the truths about my father that I told publicly and that I will continue to tell. My father started drinking heavily at age fifteen, he suffered from alcoholism his whole life, and his drinking was the primary cause of his death. Furthermore, his greatest achievements came from a decade-long stretch during which he sobered up. I speculate that he could have accomplished even more had he not abused alcohol.

Still, I will not label my father as an alcoholic. I understand that he qualified for a diagnosis of alcoholism. But that diagnosis, accurate as it was in some contexts, never defined him. I feel the same way about his depression. I understand he qualified for some sort of diagnosis, but the label "depressed" is unimportant. Such labels are harmful, not because they are false, exactly, but because their focus is misplaced.

I am at peace because there is nothing to hide. And I hope my family's story gives a glimpse into a healthy family response to the symptoms of intergenerational sickness.

Now, let's talk about a group that is unhealthy. There are three levels to every sick family: (1) the sickness itself, (2) the symptoms, and (3) the family's response to those symptoms. The family's response is sometimes even worse than the symptoms themselves. Negative family responses rely on labeling an individual. Once the individual is labeled, the intergenerational family sickness is ignored while its roots grow deeper and stronger.

The next three stories illustrate these points about the family's response and labeling individuals.

Label #1: The Bastard

The first story is about my friend Merrick, whose mother, Agatha, was sixteen and unmarried when she gave birth. Merrick is a good bit older than I am, and at the time he was born, there was a strong stigma around kids born out of wedlock. He suffered under that stigma, which he could never avoid because his father wasn't around to raise him.

But let's back up and address the family sickness, and that means talking about Agatha's family. The family featured a controlling patriarch, a self-interested mother, and several siblings. The father always tried to control who his kids would marry or date. Well, he tried to control everything, but in particular he tried to control his children's relationships. Naturally, his attempts often backfired. The eldest daughter dated a young man who was so offensive to her parents that they told her to never see him again. She married him, of course. The brother rebelled often, standing up to the patriarch in vicious, aggressive arguments. He got deep into drugs and later even attempted suicide. Then Agatha ran off with her brother's best friend, and the patriarch hired a private investigator to find them. They had gone halfway across the country, and Merrick's future father was dealing drugs.

Needless to say, the patriarch's controlling behavior was unhealthy. But his behavior was often ignored because, throughout the family's history, one or another of the siblings was always labeled as the problem. First, it was the eldest daughter who wanted to marry a guy who looked like a vagabond. Then there was the son who was labeled as a rebel. The second daughter, whom I did not mention earlier, wanted to marry a guy from a different religion. Agatha ran off and disappeared, so she was labeled as crazy. The parents focused on each disappointing child, one at a time, trying to solve the problem. It never worked. Every time they seemed to regain control of one of their kids, a new symptom of the family sickness popped up in a different sibling. It was an endless cycle of frustration.

The siblings weren't the only ones who got branded. When Agatha became pregnant, Merrick was labeled a bastard. The label was used before he was even born, by those in the family who were jealous of Agatha and also by extended family members who viewed the patriarch as competition. By branding Merrick as a bastard, they could make the patriarch look like he had failed as a father.

This process was not even connected to Merrick's immediate nuclear family, and in any case, Merrick hadn't even been born yet! He obviously couldn't have done anything to deserve a mark of shame. And yet he carried the "bastard" tag with him his whole life, and it was used against him whenever anyone had a conflict with him for any reason.

After my father's funeral, Merrick told me how validating it was to hear that my father grew up in a single-parent family. My father was a hero, and Merrick got to witness a story in which being raised by a single mother was a source of honor, not shame.

The attempt to degrade Merrick was always unacceptable and disturbing. His mother and her siblings displayed symptoms of a sick family, so it was always possible to come up with an excuse as to why their labels could apply. But shaming Merrick was just the family response to those symptoms in its purest form—because he was innocent. He couldn't have done anything to deserve the label he got, but that's how the family responded anyway.

If you were to ask anyone in a one-on-one conversation if they thought Merrick was innocent, of course they would say yes. And yet the response was still there, a response no individual would agree with. The process wasn't thought out. It was just a reaction that happened almost by instinct—not an individual instinct but the group's instinct.

Labeling and shaming Merrick allowed the group to ignore the family sickness. The irony is that Merrick's innocence made him the perfect scapegoat because it wasn't even necessary to fabricate a symptom or blow one out of proportion. Furthermore, his position in the family tree wasn't going to change no matter what. So he could be scapegoated for just existing, and he never needed to be replaced with a new scapegoat. His innocence made him the easiest target for the family's misguided response to its own symptoms.

Label #2: The Slut

This next story starts cheerfully enough. I've played music ever since I was ten. In my early twenties I started a band in which I sang and played drums at the same time. I'm sure it was all quite impressive, but it was also taxing. After a decade or so, my band members and I decided I should be a front person, so we'd use a drum machine. It was great, but I had a problem. I just stood in front of the audience like a statue, singing.

I realized it was time I learned how to dance, so I watched tutorials on the internet and practiced at home. It wasn't enough, though, and after a few months, I mustered the courage to attend local street dance events. Aaron, one of the first people I met at those events, was an excellent competitor who often taught others in the scene. He offered to train me, and I gladly accepted the offer. At first, it was the happiest time of my life. I was coming out of a deep depression, and dance felt like the perfect way to end that unhappy phase of my life.

Here is where the story stops being cheerful. After a few years, I noticed Aaron's strange behavior toward women and girls. In particular, he showed way too much attention to a female dancer, Olivia, who was only fourteen years old. I don't think this young girl had ever met her father, she had a troubled relationship with her mother, and she was looking for a way out of her miserable day-to-day life. Dance seemed to provide that path. Aaron convinced her he could make her a successful dancer, that he could be her teacher and coach.

But he wanted to be more than just her coach, and he was in his late twenties while she was fourteen. He manipulated her into a sexual relationship, which wouldn't have exactly met the standards of consent even if she were old enough. He convinced her he would push her dance career in return for sex, and he also fed her a whole lot of lies about marrying her when she turned eighteen.

So far, this might sound like an ugly but simple story of an older male preying on a young girl. And if Aaron and Olivia had been the only two people involved, then that would have been the whole story. But the tale becomes more disturbing, nightmarish even, when it includes the various families involved and how they responded.

To explain the family response, I must describe the grooming process that allowed Aaron to prey on this young girl. Karin, Aaron's girlfriend at the time, was his primary accomplice. But she wasn't the only accomplice. The girl's own mother helped as well! And Aaron was not the first adult male the mother had tried to groom her daughter for. There had been a previous dance teacher, Cedric, who did not acquiesce to the grooming of his student. Cedric was just trying to be Olivia's dance teacher. But the mother didn't understand or didn't care.

I'll never forget a text Olivia's mother sent me when the whole sordid story became public. She wrote, "And here I thought Aaron was a man of morals, like Cedric, who would wait until Olivia turned eighteen."

Now you know the mother's definition of a "man of morals." I won't go into further detail about how the mother groomed her own daughter, because that's enough information for you to understand why the family's response was so traumatic.

Olivia knew her family's response would be a problem, so she initially lied about the relationship. Aaron encouraged her to lie, and he even coached her on how to lie effectively.

But Aaron was eventually exposed because of other sexual misbehavior. That girlfriend, Karin? Well, Aaron impregnated her and then dumped her. As a response, Karin started dating Aaron's worst enemy in the dance scene—a physically abusive man named Billy—who had a long history of threatening people with knives, guns, and crowbars.

Well, Billy hated Aaron, and he was close friends with Cedric. So Cedric and Billy got together, and they realized Olivia was lying about Aaron. Billy and Karin then conned Olivia into going out to dinner with them. They got her hopped up on drugs and tried to manipulate her into discussing her relationship with Aaron. When that didn't work, they threatened her with a gun.

Even those threats failed, so Cedric, Billy, and Karin approached Olivia's mother. They convinced her that Olivia needed to be punished for her behavior. So one day, while Olivia was napping on a couch, Cedric, Billy, and Karin woke her up and verbally attacked her. I don't know everything that was said, but in texts to me afterward, they told me Olivia was a slut and a disgusting liar. They said she had embarrassed them and that she "needs to learn to keep her legs closed." They told me they would make sure she never danced again.

Olivia's mother joined in on the slut-shaming, sending me long messages discussing Olivia's inability to make good decisions, her terrible taste in men, and her sexual immorality. (I can't imagine where she might have learned all that from.) The mother decided Olivia needed to be punished, so she banned her from dancing and took away her artistic opportunities. This was all particularly stinging for Olivia, who had complied with Aaron's sexual desires only because she thought doing so would further her dance career.

This is how Olivia got labeled a "slut," a label that followed her long after her mother relented and allowed her to dance again. The wider dance community continued to shame her, and in some cases, to even shame people who associated with her. Several families were involved, including the smallest unit, Olivia and her mother, and extending out to eventually include an entire dance scene. Every single one of Olivia's families failed her, from the smallest to the largest. None offered an acceptable response to what were, in her case, mere symptoms of intergenerational family sickness.

But what about Aaron? This guy was not innocent, and he was not just displaying symptoms. He was sick. He was an actual predator. What happened to him?

He too was labeled, and I would argue he deserved the label of sexual predator. In fact, I did everything I could to persuade Olivia to go with me to the police so he would be prosecuted and, well, labeled. Looking at it as a legal matter, I thought he should carry that sex offender tag around so he could not teach again. But Olivia wouldn't talk to the police because of her mother's involvement in the grooming process.

The dance scene, though, labeled Aaron a predator. The dance family pursued a sort of social media justice. At first, it seemed like Aaron deserved it, and I didn't interfere. But maybe I should have, because I later learned of enormous problems.

Karin, Aaron's ex-girlfriend, was not only an accomplice. Karin had raped one of my friends and sexually assaulted at least two others. She had a history of sexual misbehavior with underage boys as well as a history of domestic violence that included assault with a deadly weapon. Given my experience with troubled couples, I would suggest that the primary reason Aaron and Karin ever got together was that they were both predatory. Similarly, the primary reason Billy and Karin got together was probably that they were both abusive.

More layers of intergenerational family sickness were uncovered. Aaron had another ex-girlfriend who was his accomplice in a previous teaching position. Before becoming Aaron's enemy, Billy had helped Aaron attempt to groom another teenage girl, although it's unclear whether Billy realized what Aaron was up to. So of course Billy, Karin, and Aaron's other ex-girlfriend were Aaron's social media accusers, painting a picture of Aaron as the "Bill Cosby of the dance scene."

But, as it turns out, Aaron wasn't a solo predator. He was part of an entire group of people who were abusive or predatory, and they all groomed one another to behave that way. I can't pretend I know everything, but I eventually learned that at least a dozen people were in this group. The group had been instrumental in creating the dance scene, so the wider family that slut-shamed Olivia was sick from the roots up, just like her immediate family was sick.

Aaron had several accomplices, and many wanted Aaron to be the fall guy so they could sweep their own misbehavior under the rug. But focusing on individuals who had something to hide misses the point that whole groups had something to hide. Entire families were involved in this mess. So even labeling Aaron a predator, a label he deserved, still covered up the family sickness for several different groups.

I want to make it clear that there can be sick individuals, and there are even times when an individual should be labeled. Aaron is one clear case. But even in those rare, specific cases, the labeling process can still hide the family sickness. So whenever you see an individual being scapegoated, be careful.

And how about Olivia? The way she was labeled served no purpose other than to cover up the real problems. I want to bring up a few points about that "slut" label Olivia had to carry.

Eventually, Karin was labeled the same way. But Karin was not a slut. She was abusive and had committed sexual assaults. That weird equivalence of calling both Oliva and Karin "sluts" was based on tired societal stereotypes; the labels themselves were offensive and misleading.

Olivia once told me, "You know, I can't figure out what's worse, that Aaron had sex with me or that Billy ambushed me while I was sleeping on the couch." Well, Olivia, from the outside looking in, I can't figure it out either. I can't tell which caused more trauma—Aaron's sexual assaults or the whole family's relentless attempts to shame Olivia for his criminal acts.

Label #3: The Golden Child

This story is about a business I did consulting for. The business was owned by a man who envied other people's successes, but who had no vision for what his business should be in its own right. So he was kind of always chasing after the next big thing. He was always unhappy, which is a defining characteristic of those who succumb to jealousy.

When I started working with the business, I noticed the owner had a favorite employee—his chief strategist, Mark. In some ways, it seemed Mark was everything the owner wasn't. Mark was technologically savvy and detail oriented. He approached every question from the perspective of finding a mathematical system to deal with the issue. As far as anyone could tell, Mark's systems were successful.

So at first, Mark was my main point of contact. Then, suddenly, it seemed no one in the business wanted to associate with him. I couldn't figure out what had happened. I kept hearing all sorts of talk about his depression and his mental illness. There were claims that he couldn't be considered reliable because of these issues. It didn't quite make sense, though. Everyone said he was doing the job he was supposed to do. And yet there was endless chatter about his mental health and then about his supposedly deteriorating marriage.

I remember when the owner told me, "You better watch out for Mark. He's a sick, sick man." I was shocked. Mark had been, as far as I could tell, second in command at the business. An article about the firm had just been published in a trade magazine, and Mark was featured on the cover with the owner's family.

I never learned why the owner turned on Mark. But Mark was bullied out of the business, and his alleged mental illness was the reason.

As soon as Mark left, the owner had a new favorite—Mary, the head salesperson. Well, actually, Mary was the only person making sales other than the boss, although others were trying to learn that role. She also had the longest tenure of any employee, so it wasn't surprising that her accomplishments were praised.

But then the owner turned on Mary too. It seemed somewhat justifiable since Mary had blown up at other employees a couple of times and had had a few dramatic shouting matches with the owner himself. Mary was labeled "crazy," which didn't seem too out of line if you focused on those big events. But in my work with her, Mary had always been professional, courteous, and diligent. So I had a hard time reconciling the person that I heard about with the person I worked with.

However, at this juncture, I was working remotely with the firm. I wasn't there every day. I liked the owner; he was charismatic, optimistic, and ambitious. So I gave him the benefit of the doubt, even when Mary was driven out of the business as well.

The next employee the owner favored, though, raised some suspicions. This guy, Christopher, never struck me as much of a talent. He was a close friend of the owner's son. Other than that, he just seemed like a regular employee, and that is fine. But why, other than his friendship, was he the new "employee of the month"?

Christopher's tenure at the top of the totem pole didn't last long. Soon he was labeled "stupid" and "incompetent." I never saw any evidence to back up those labels, though, other than that Christopher was thrown into roles he wasn't yet prepared for. When he got the proper training, he performed well.

And anyway, a new golden child, Simon, was now being groomed to be a CEO type, almost a replacement for the owner. Simon had impeccable credentials, not to mention a fantastic set of suits and ties. Simon spoke, acted, and dressed like a top manager. The owner even told me, "Simon is going to save this business." I enjoyed working with Simon, and I felt that with him at the helm and the owner's total support, the business was finally ready to turn the corner.

Then that all changed. Once again, no one wanted to associate with the former golden child. I remember vividly a meeting in which everyone avoided even sitting next to him. He was labeled a "narcissist" and called "selfish" and "manipulative." The same habits everyone had once praised were turned into objects of ridicule. Simon was soon fired.

At this point, I knew the business was in deep trouble. I started creating my exit strategy from the consulting contract. But before I left, I got to see one more golden child get turned into a scapegoat. Eric, another planner, somewhat similar to Mark, had been my closest friend at the company. He was brilliant, and after Simon left, the owner lavished praise on Eric. Eric had created an incredible spreadsheet detailing all the firm's clients and what they were paying. The fee structure was disorganized and inefficient. The firm could increase profits by normalizing the way it collected fees, even if some clients left. I was amazed. This kid was the kind of employee I imagined any owner would dream of having. And the owner did seem impressed at first. But a shadow came across his face. He turned to Eric and said, "And how do you have so much spare time to do all this?" Sure enough, Eric was labeled "lazy" and "unproductive." By now, the process was familiar. Eric was being forced out.

A week after Eric left, I had a meeting with the boss. He told me he was so impressed with my work. He even said he had always known that someday I would be the one to save the business.

I resigned, obviously.

After leaving, I learned about one more employee who was transformed from golden child into scapegoat. Mika was a technology specialist, and no one ever criticized his work. It seems he was fired because the owner's girlfriend didn't like him and labeled him "weird."

Anyway, a couple of years after I left, regulators sanctioned the business because of the owner's outright illegal behavior. He had been defrauding clients. He had to pay some huge fines. The business wasn't shut down, but it was tricky there for a few months. So there's the family sickness—the organizational dysfunction in a nutshell.

Now let's talk about all the individual employees who were labeled. Mark, who was labeled mentally ill, got a job teaching computer programming and music at a community college. Mary, the supposedly crazy one, went to work at an insurance firm and soon doubled her take-home pay. Simon, the so-called narcissist, became vice president of a college. Eric, the alleged lazy one, became a planner for another firm at a higher salary. And Mika? Well, his career took off the moment he left the firm.

Every employee who was forced out became more successful. The one employee who remained unsuccessful and unhappy was Christopher—the only former golden child unfortunate enough to keep his job. Other employees who stuck around also suffered—like the receptionist who cried herself to sleep every night because of the owner's mood swings. Another receptionist couldn't sleep at all. Both women blamed themselves for what were symptoms of a sick family.

But they weren't to blame. Look at the labeled individuals, who were all better off once they left the dysfunctional work family. Meanwhile, the sick business stayed sick. It stayed sick even after the owner left and handed over the business to his kids. When the business was finally, mercifully sold, the new firm was paying for what was pretty much just a client list.

The business always had deep organizational problems due to a controlling founder who had no clear purpose other than envy. The business was unhealthy from the beginning, sick from the top down. Just before he was fired, Simon told me, "I've worked in some real shitholes before. But I've never seen a firm like this where there is just no sense of how to move forward."

This is an excellent example of a few important principles. First, it shows the problem with labeling individuals even when those labels are accurate in some contexts. I got to know Mark well, and the truth is that he was depressed. But that doesn't matter in the context of the unhealthy organization, because questions about that label's accuracy were misguided in the first place. The question should have been, "Why are we discussing his mental health at all?" He was doing a good job, so it was an inappropriate and unacceptable topic for office gossip.

Outside of a sick family, people don't get scapegoated or shamed for mental health issues. Even if Mark was depressed, no one at the business was a qualified therapist. A qualified therapist would never diagnose a man based on one symptom or by observing him in only one setting. So the fact that the label turned out to be accurate was just a coincidence.

All of the other negative labels were either inaccurate or too vague to be evaluated. But the second principle this story illustrates is that even positive labels can be harmful because they focus too much on the individual while ignoring the group dynamic. A business is sick if employees are always either praised for being perfect or trashed for being worthless, with no room for complex gray areas. And even if the golden children never become scapegoats, it's still problematic to elevate an employee to the status of savior, because it reflects poorly on everyone else. If this one employee is so great, so integral to the firm's success, then what does that say about how other staffers are valued?

Positive labels have unintended negative consequences because they put an individual into a fixed mindset. For example, I was labeled "smart." Now, I'd rather be labeled smart than be labeled stupid. The problem is if I'm smart, then how can I be wrong? This is a big issue because I cannot succeed as an entrepreneur without taking calculated risks, and some of those risks aren't going to work out. The sooner I admit I'm wrong and change course, the sooner I can become successful. But it's hard to admit that I'm wrong when I care about living up to the label of being smart.

When a family is sick, labeling individuals always strengthens the family sickness—whether the labels are positive or negative. Each time an individual gets labeled, it sets them up to be removed and replaced. And every time one individual is replaced, a new individual steps into the same role. But the new individual has less experience in the group, fewer connections, and thus less influence. While the role itself becomes more powerful, the new individual has less power than their predecessor did. The group itself gains even more influence, but all the remaining individuals have just a little bit less influence.

Every time a family labels and replaces an individual, the ability of any remaining individual to influence the family declines. As time goes on, the potential influence of individuals, no matter how remarkable they may be, drops to nothing. This is so much more obvious in businesses than in other types of families because even the healthiest business hires and fires. Businesses replace people all the time. Whether the business is healthy or unhealthy, every new hire has just a little bit less power compared to the organization as a whole. So in unhealthy businesses, the people come and go, but the dysfunction remains.

Four Principles

The three previous stories illustrate four important principles about most sick families.

1. Addressing mere symptoms doesn't work. In a sick family, whenever one symptom recedes, a new symptom pops up somewhere else.
2. The family assigns a label to the member with the most attention-grabbing symptom. The labeling process is often misguided, inaccurate, and offensive.

3. The labeling process, no matter how accurate, focuses on an individual and allows the family sickness to be ignored, minimized, or enabled.
4. Shame surrounding the labeling process creates emotional trauma that can be even worse than the symptoms.

I've noticed some other factors in the labeling process. In today's society, labeling often seems authoritative or reasonable because people use (or misuse) psychiatric terms to label others: codependence, narcissism, borderline personality disorder, depression, autism, social anxiety, and so on. But the medical terms don't make labeling less harmful. Furthermore, people often use terms loaded with politics or religion when labeling others. Family members feel as though they might be tarred by the same insults if they don't join in on blaming the scapegoat.

I want to be careful here because I talk a lot about scapegoating. However, sometimes we label people in ways that are harmful, even though it doesn't look like scapegoating. It might even look like compassion.

For instance, take autism, which is a diagnosis that applies to me. I have no problem being autistic. I don't even mind the label, and I often apply it to myself. But I'm glad the label autistic wasn't in common use when I was growing up. As a kid, I was not diagnosed with autism or any other condition.

I didn't talk to people until I was about ten years old, so most people thought I was strange. And at age five or six, I was obsessed with unusual activities such as copying the periodic table of the elements from the dictionary, inventing my own numbering systems (I was a big fan of base-12 systems), and learning all I could about trapezoids and parallelograms.

Oh, and dinosaurs—can't forget the dinosaurs.

But I never thought of myself as abnormal or even unusual. I just figured most people didn't talk about their obsessions with trapezoids. I mean, I never did. Of course, that was because I didn't talk at all.

Anyway, while reading through an internet forum, I came across a comment by someone who identified himself as autistic. He was unhappy because another forum member had been commenting about reading people's facial cues in a video. He wrote, "Since I'm autistic, I can't do that." This poor guy—somebody who thought they were being compassionate toward the neuro-divergent told him he's autistic, and now he thinks the label defines him.

I wanted to tell him, "Hey, you can learn. That's kind of what we autistic people are good at—learning in a very focused and, frankly, obsessive way. Regardless of autism or any genetic conditions, you can learn about social cues and nonverbal communication just like you can learn about ptero-dactyls and Pythagoras. In fact, if you want to, you can learn how to present a facade of empathy, other various normal emotions, and all the other stuff that many people like to see." I did that. It was useful. In fact I found it was necessary in order to make a steady living.

But if someone believes strongly in their "autistic" label, they won't learn those social skills. It doesn't fit the definition, so they become the label.

I hope most people who label a kid autistic do so because they are trying to help other people understand the young person. And you know what? When presented properly, the label might do its job. In some contexts, a label like "autistic" can help other people understand the child who comes off as different and whose behavior seems so inexplicable. But you have to be careful because there are serious unintended consequences if the child internalizes the label. And there are much worse labels than "autistic."

Kent A. Kiehl, author of *The Psychopath Whisperer: The Science of Those Without Conscience*, is considered one of the world's primary authorities on psychopaths. Dr. Kiehl is adamant that no young person should ever be diagnosed as a psychopath. He has run into so many people who were improperly labeled as kids, and they started acting like psychopaths as soon as they got slapped with that label.

I hope it is clear why I am so concerned about how families respond to symptoms. You can influence someone's behavior to be psychopathic just by labeling the person a "psychopath." So what else do you think you can push people into by slapping a label on them?

And yes, the same applies to labels you tag yourself with. According to some therapists I talk with, there is an unusual increase in the number of people who want to be labeled or diagnosed. At first, it was people wanting to be diagnosed with anxiety or depression, and this makes some sense because with a diagnosis, the patient could get treatment. But recently a therapist told me how disturbing it was to deal with a patient who demanded to be diagnosed with borderline personality disorder.

I don't know where this is coming from, but I do know many of us label ourselves in our own heads. When we label ourselves, we perpetuate family sickness and even spread that sickness by accepting it as normal or correct. I think about this all the time because I've done prison ministry for years, working with so many people who experienced incarceration. Most of them were labeled long before they could possibly have done anything to deserve the labels they were stuck with.

Labeling Is Never Compassionate

I want to further explore the negative effects of labeling, because so many people believe it's somehow helpful to diagnose others or themselves. Mental illness is another condition for which people often think they are being compassionate by labeling someone.

As I mentioned in the introduction, I used to hallucinate constantly, and I suffered from long bouts of paranoia. When confronted with someone like me, many people respond by diagnosing the condition. They give it a name such as schizophrenia. They try to convince me to label myself the same way. Finally, they use the diagnosis, the name, to explain my behavior. "Oh, you act that way because you are schizophrenic."

This is wrong and entirely backward. Mental health diagnoses do not explain someone's behavior. In fact, someone's behavior is supposed to lead to the diagnosis! No one acts a certain way because of a mental illness or personality disorder. It's the other way around—the way someone acts convinces a psychiatrist to apply the diagnosis.

Many mental health issues, besides being mere symptoms of family sickness, perhaps should be viewed more as signals than symptoms. Think about physical pain for a moment. Of course I don't want to be in pain, but if I injure myself the pain does serve as a warning, alerting me that my body needs healing. If I never experienced any pain, I could end up dead of an injury I was never even aware of. Similarly, negative emotions such as anxiety and depression are sometimes flashing lights alerting us to dangers.

At times in my life, depression helped me because I recognized it as a signal that I was choosing to stay in toxic relationships or groups. But when I received those signals, too often I tried to squash them. It was as if I were to deal with the warning lights on my car's dashboard by smashing them with a sledgehammer. Now some people prefer the method of taping a piece of paper over the red light so they don't have to look at it, but either way, the warning isn't the problem.

One more aspect of the labeling process is worth discussing. Sometimes, the family member getting labeled is the least healthy member of the family. Sometimes, just sometimes, the scapegoat is the sickest member, and the family tries to be compassionate or empathetic. But even in such situations, the sick family member is always codependent. They convince the rest of the family that in order to function, they need this or that from everyone else. So the empathy shown by everyone else allows the least healthy, most dependent member to control the whole family.

Their codependence requires everyone's attention and makes growth impossible. The family is engaged in constant crisis management. Everyone is very empathetic, and no one sets effective boundaries. Family members get to feel better about themselves by thinking they are being compassionate toward the least healthy one, who, as "everyone knows," can't manage to do anything for themselves. It is precisely that belief—spawned from the labeling process—that makes growth impossible. The sickest, most codependent members *can* do something for themselves, but everyone else in the family labels and enables instead.

Growth Hurts at First

Bad romantic relationships often end up in this state of codependence. Codependent relationships have an inherent stability because both partners agree to put up with each other's messes. In return, they don't have to be alone, and they don't have to deal with the pain of growth.

Growth almost always hurts. Setting boundaries causes short-term pain. Real healing, whether physical, emotional, or spiritual, causes discomfort at first. That's why it's so important to remember that symptoms are not the sickness. When you start to heal, the symptoms often get worse for a time. Things are changing, so now the family is stressed.

If symptoms are severe, they might have to be dealt with directly, just like I had to take an anesthetic when I got my wisdom teeth pulled. Sometimes painkillers are necessary. For instance, I would never suggest that someone quit using antidepressants if those drugs seem to work. Even though the placebo effect is real, and even though it might not even be the drug that's doing the work, if the mere belief in the drug's effectiveness helps you feel better, then by all means, keep believing. Yes, your depression may be a mere symptom of a deeper family illness. But then again, you might need to stabilize your emotions first before dealing with that reality.

However, painkillers alone won't heal sickness. I took an anesthetic when I got my wisdom teeth pulled, but I didn't expect the anesthetic to heal my jaw. In the same way, you can't expect painkillers like antidepressants to heal intergenerational sickness.

In the following chapter, we'll look at how to heal a sick family. But I want to share one more story to summarize these first two chapters. Ever since I was a teenager, I've had gut problems. When the COVID-19 lockdown hit, I decided I was going to get something from the situation. I was going to figure out what was up with my digestion, once and for all. And I did it. I discovered the diet that works for me.

Then one day, right before eating, I was playing a *Star*

Wars game on my phone. I'm in a small guild of people who don't take the game too seriously. Suddenly, a player named Victory rejoined the guild. Now this "Victory" guy is someone who does take the game seriously—way too seriously. He had joined the guild a few times in the past, and always quit in anger when he didn't get his way. Of course, not only did he quit, but he also spread so much gossip, anxiety, and resentment over whatever argument he was having that other people quit too. The moment Victory rejoined the guild, he demanded he be made an officer. Thankfully, the guild leader kicked him out instead. As it turns out, this video game guild was a fairly healthy family!

Anyway, I brought up that stuff about my gut because I became physically ill when I saw that Victory was trying to return to the gaming group, which I don't even care much about. My indigestion was worse than when I spent an entire day eating nothing but pizza and ice cream. Folks, this is a trivial online video game. But a brief encounter with an emotionally abusive person affected my health that much.

All right. Let's move on to healing.

CHAPTER 3

HOW TO START HEALING A SICK FAMILY

Fortunately, healing a sick family does not require the ability to perfectly distinguish between sickness, symptoms, and the response to symptoms. Instead, healing starts whenever any family member, regardless of their position or status, stops participating in the cycle of sickness. You can start the healing process by staying connected to the other family members while refusing to take sides in their conflicts with each other.

I ONCE CAME ACROSS AN INTERNET MEME THAT POSited the following dilemma: "You meet your eighteen-year-old self. You can say only three words. What do you say?"

My answer? "Don't take sides."

Or as an older and much wiser pastor once remarked to me, "If the bullet doesn't have your name on it, get out of its way." If I could teach one lesson to my eighteen-year-old self, that would be it. When I look at my biggest mistakes, I realize that taking sides in other people's conflicts is at the root of most of those mistakes. And in some troubled families I've worked with, refusing to take sides has led to more healing than everything else combined.

Don't Take Sides

For several reasons, I don't take sides in other peoples' conflicts. The first is simple: I have no way of knowing what really happened.

In fact, because memory is unreliable, the people in the conflict may not even know what really happened. On top of that, because of cognitive bias, if I take sides, I accept information that agrees with my stance while ignoring or minimizing information that contradicts it. I will support the side I took during times when, if I were a neutral observer, I would have a different opinion. So even if I'm not being manipulated, I will essentially manipulate myself. That's what I call "the information issue," but there are deeper reasons why I should not take sides.

We all act differently under conditions of conflict. Also, all of us act differently behind closed doors as compared to how we act in public. Further, most of us act at least a little bit differently toward those who have more power or status than we do, compared to those who are equals or those who have less. Finally, most people act differently toward others depending on the type of relationship. Strangers, our social circle, close friends, romantic partners, parents or ancestors, children, and cousins or siblings may all get disparate treatment.

This means that no matter how well I think I know someone, I might not know how they are acting in a conflict. If I take a side, I may very well be supporting someone who is being abusive, acting unethically, or using me in ways I don't understand.

Also, just because there is a bad guy doesn't mean there is a good guy. Real life is not like the movies. More conflicts feature two bad guys than feature a hero and a villain. Sure, perhaps one bad guy is not quite as awful as the other bad guy. But if you take sides, you may find yourself stuck with an ally you'd be better off without. You may find out, at great cost and emotional agony, that your new ally is worse than an enemy.

Furthermore, taking sides can harm your relationship with the person whose side you took! When in conflict, people often regress. They think in terms of winning and losing, not in terms of compassion, shared goals, or even their own best interests. And they often stay in that win-or-lose mindset regardless of whether or not it makes sense.

This is why taking sides as a peacemaker so often backfires. Trying to encourage or manipulate someone who is deep in conflict, even if you think you are leading them in the right direction, can easily turn into a contest about winning and losing because they are stuck in an aggressive mindset. They don't want to lose, so they resist your suggestions, just because the suggestion is coming from someone else and not them.

I used to be quite naive about abusive relationships. I thought that if a friend was in an abusive relationship, I should encourage them to leave. *Nope.* Such encouragement often strengthens the resolve of the victim to stay in the relationship, partly because they don't want to experience what feels like a loss. And losing can mean any number of things. The victim might not want to admit to others that they were wrong about the relationship, they may not want to be perceived as a failure, or they may not want to lose their abuser to someone else.

Depending on the severity of the abuse, the victim might

just be afraid. Even worse, since abusers are excellent at playing the victim, the actual victim may feel that I am advocating some form of revenge by encouraging them to leave. At that point, the victim feels guilty, which drives the victim back to the abuser. Now the abuser has become even more powerful (and is suspicious of and perhaps angry at me).

It doesn't get any better in a mutually abusive relationship. Say two of my friends are in an abusive relationship with each other, and they are both acting out in toxic ways. Trying to "help" them stay together and improve their relationship only pushes me to take one side or another in their arguments. This is true in a non-abusive relationship as well. Trying to "help" pushes me to accidentally end up on someone's side in an argument, putting the other person on the defensive.

No, by far the best decision is to not take sides and instead be friends with each person so that neither gets isolated. It's also important to model non-abusive behavior. I don't waste a lot of time telling people to stop being abusive. I mostly just act non-abusively.

Abuse is often based on the mindset that people are either all bad or all good, with no in-between. The reality that we are all a mix of good and bad qualities is ignored. This extreme mindset, which is often called "splitting," is a big part of why abusers so often blame others. They can't admit to being even a little bit wrong or else they feel they are all wrong. This mindset says that everything is always their partner's fault.

When I refuse to take sides, I am modeling non-abusive behavior. I am showing, not telling, that people are a mix of good qualities and bad. Or I am modeling that people's qualities don't need to be categorized as good or bad. Either approach is effective.

When members of a group or family have conflicts with

one another, dragging others into the conflict results in the worst type of escalation. If two people have a conflict with each other, then it is possible for just the two of them to reach a resolution. No one else needs to be involved. But from the moment someone else enters the conflict—even as an intended peacemaker or a voice of reason—in that instant, the conflict can no longer be resolved without the participation of all three people. This can potentially still work if both people requested the participation of a neutral third party who refuses to take sides. But if the third person is biased toward one side, then the one in the minority will likely seek an ally as well.

If too many people are involved in the conflict, then a resolution becomes impossible. The conflict grows exponentially. In a two-person conflict, only one resolution is necessary—the one between the two people. In a three-person conflict, four resolutions are necessary—one resolution each for the three pairs, plus a resolution for the three-person group as a whole. In a four-person conflict, as many as ten resolutions may be necessary: a resolution for each of the six possible pairings of people, plus resolutions for each trio, and also a resolution for the entire four-person group. Once five people are involved in the conflict, it becomes far too complex sheerly on a mathematical level.

This is why I say peacemongers—folks who seem to genuinely believe the best way to deal with any conflict is to try to smooth things over—are often nearly as toxic in group settings as are outright abusers. Peacemongers enlist the aid of other members in the group to calm people down. They deliver messages to and from members, playing a game of telephone that replaces one-on-one communication. They attempt to force people to like one another. They ignore divisions in the hope that the conflicts will magically disappear. They try to make everyone get along without ever letting anyone express how they actually feel. Almost every member of the group eventually ends up being involved, so the conflict becomes too complex to resolve.

The human mind doesn't like that level of complexity. So as the conflict escalates, people regress into the violence-based mindset of only two sides.

One truth about physical violence is that, once violence starts, no matter how many sides there once were, the number of factions always gets reduced to two. It's hard enough to avoid friendly fire even when there are only allies and enemies. During physical violence, the chaos and confusion probably makes multiple sides impossible. Once physical violence breaks out, all involved typically end up on one side or the other.

When interpersonal conflicts escalate as others join the mix, the violence mindset takes over. Everyone involved typically takes one of only two sides. The general mentality becomes, "My side is good, and the other side is evil." When that happens, activities that should be either harmless or beneficial to team building become destructive instead. Consider gossip, which normally helps people bond. But if people take sides in an escalating conflict, gossip becomes a tool for each faction to demonize the other.

Stay Out of It

Now let's consider a behavioral pattern that is even worse than taking sides. Let's look at what happens if you try to control anyone's relationship to someone else.

In short, it's going to blow up in your face. If you forbid

your kid from dating someone, they'll probably marry them. If you try to bring together two people who aren't interested, they may end up hating each other.

Even if you succeed in manipulating people for a while, there is another problem. If you try to control anyone's relationship with someone else, you will end up with some of the stress, anxiety, and resentment of their relationship. And anytime you try to control someone else's relationship to an issue, idea, goal, or problem, you take on some of the stress that should be theirs.

I'd bet that everyone reading this has experienced that in their own lives. As far back as childhood, if you tried to take emotional responsibility for your parents' relationship, you likely absorbed some of their tension and stress. So you may already perceive the negative consequences of controlling behavior.

Even if you do not want to be controlling, though, people will often try to drag you into their relationship with something or someone else. This is because lots of people would love to give you power or control so they can avoid responsibility.

For instance, when someone asks for your advice about their relationship with an intimate partner, watch out. I adamantly refuse to give dating advice, and for good reason. People aren't looking for advice when they talk to me about their significant other. They're looking for an ally. If I'm foolish enough to become one, I will take on the stress of their relationship.

Every time I've had a goal that wasn't well thought out, I tried to convince someone else to help me achieve that goal. Whether or not I consciously realized it, I wanted other people to join me in my quest because they'd share some of the stress that should be all mine. When my goals are clear and worthwhile, I don't need to *convince* anyone to do anything.

They often enthusiastically say yes. Actually, they sometimes volunteer before I can even ask.

The reverse situation is similar. When someone asks me to do something and I feel like saying no, usually that feeling occurs because the other person is trying to drag me into a relationship I ought to stay out of—usually their relationship with another person. But sometimes people try to drag me into their relationship with their own ideas, problems, issues, or goals. Either way, I will end up with more anxiety and they will end up with less responsibility, so we both suffer.

Let's apply this to a real-world question that a young woman recently asked me: "How do I know the difference between enabling someone and supporting them as they try to change?" This is where self-help works. When you feel anxiety, you are enabling. When you feel resentment, it means you are saying yes when you ought to say no.

This is also a great example of when symptoms are actually beneficial signals. Believe it or not, anxiety and resentment aren't always negative emotions. Any common human emotion must serve some positive purpose under some set of circumstances, or else it wouldn't continue to exist. Anxiety and resentment serve as excellent signals that boundaries are being violated. Pay attention to those signals instead of blaming yourself for feeling bad, and the emotional environment surrounding you will begin to change.

If You Want to Say No, That's a Good Enough Reason to Say No

Let's discuss changing your emotional environment. For many people, the first and most important step is learning to say no when you want to say no, while remaining connected to other people.

It was so simple for me to say, "Anytime I want to say no, I will say no." But it was not so easy to follow through with saying no when people looked at me with puppy dog eyes. It was hard to say no when friends made reasonable requests that took me off guard. I needed a conceptual framework to help me understand how to say no while remaining connected to the group.

Triangles

I visualize relationships as triangles. Each person is one point of the triangle. One of my favorite academics, sociologist Randall Collins, says, "Three is the lowest number for social structures." In other words, you can have a two-person relationship, but two people aren't quite enough to form a group, a family. A relationship that involves only two people is too volatile or unpredictable. At least one more person is needed to stabilize the group.

The key is to understand the third person's role in stabilizing the relationship. Again, imagine you and any two other people—let's say you, your father, and your mother—make a triangle. Visualize the three of you as the three points on the triangle. You are directly connected to your father and mother on two of the three sides of the triangle. Your father and mother are directly connected to each other on the third side, which does not include you.

You can affect each of the two sides of the triangle that include you. You can affect your relationship with your mother and your relationship with your father. And you can change your current relationship with either your mother, or your father, or both. But what happens if you try to control the side of the triangle that does not include you? What happens when you try to affect your parent's relationship? What happens when you see a problem with the way your parents relate to each other and then try to solve that problem?

What happens is you take on some of the stress of your parents' relationship with each other. This makes their relationship with each other less stressful, but their relationship with you becomes more stressful! Do they now have more or less incentive to address the problem in their relationship with each other? They have less incentive. On the other hand, they have more incentive to focus on their problems with you.

You've stabilized precisely the problem you were unhappy about, making it easier for your parents to tolerate the problems they have with each other. Not only have you made the triangle more stable, but you've stabilized its worst parts.

And of course, this isn't true only of you and your parents. It's true of you and any two other people.

Let's look at common ways that people unintentionally stabilize the problem they had hoped to address. One example is a series of phone conversations I witnessed between my friend Richard, his older brother, and their father. Richard lives with his mother. His older brother, who is autistic, lives with their father. Richard has told me that his father is tyrannical, abusive, and often outright narcissistic. His father is also a successful businessman.

Richard was talking with me when he got a phone message from his father. The father was raging about Richard's brother, who apparently hadn't immediately picked up the phone when the father called. The father was out of town, threatening to send a business partner to stay at the house to look after the brother. The business partner had already refused to do this, but the father didn't care.

After receiving the message, Richard called his father back

and tried to mollify him. He offered excuses for his brother's behavior, saying he was probably just playing video games. He told his father, "There is no need to go from zero to one hundred on this issue." Richard promised to talk with the brother and to persuade him to respond more quickly to their father's messages.

Then Richard called his brother. Of course, the brother promptly picked up the phone when Richard called. Richard offered reassurances: "Everyone knows you can take care of yourself. We all know you're capable. Dad just gets worried, you know? So just call him back immediately when he messages you, OK?" After that conversation ended, Richard called his father and left another message. (Notice that the father never picks up the phone when his son calls.) Richard explained that everything was now OK, that he told his brother to always pick up their phone when the father calls.

Then Richard turned to me and sheepishly told me that his father was drunk.

All right. A whole lot of bright red flags are waving here. I won't even list them all. For now, I want to focus on what happens when Richard tries to intervene in his father and brother's relationship by playing peacemaker and delivering messages.

What happens is that Richard ends up supporting his father's abuse of his brother. This is heartbreaking because the first time Richard ever talked to me about his family, he mentioned his worry about the effect his father's abuse would have on his brother. Yet here he is making it worse.

Not only that but every time he delivers a message, he takes on the stress that should be between his father and brother. At the same time, he stabilizes their abusive relationship. Their father is addicted to alcohol and totally out of control in his personal life, no matter how successful he may be in business. And like most out-of-control people, he deals with his issues by trying to control others. So here Richard is, adding to the control issues by reducing the stress his father has to experience from his own behavior! The worst part is that Richard thinks he's making things better by calming his father down, telling his brother what to do, and gossiping with them both.

His brother is twenty-two. The brother has one option available to him to end the abuse—leave the father's house. The only way that is likely to happen is if the stress of the relationship between the brother and the father remains where it belongs—between the brother and the father.

If Richard stays out of their relationship, will that stress eventually lead to a volcanic blowup by the father? Probably. Will that blowup be what finally persuades the brother to leave the house? Maybe, or maybe not. But if Richard keeps playing peacemaker, his brother will probably never leave. Richard is his brother's best friend. His brother is isolated, and he needs Richard to be a brother and a friend, not the agent of an abusive old man.

Every attempt Richard makes to manage the relationship between his brother and his father is stabilizing, reinforcing, and enabling that relationship's toxic elements, and at the same time making Richard's relationship with his family members worse.

Have you ever tried to give someone advice on how to deal with a conflict with a mutual friend and, instead of taking your advice, they get defensive and double down on their behavior? Or perhaps you have experienced the reverse. You have a conflict, someone tells you how to deal with it, and your response is some version of, "Well, what do you know?" So you try to prove them wrong. Whatever behavioral patterns they were trying to change just got stronger, and now you're pissed off at them too.

One of My Biggest Mistakes Ever

Two of my closest friends, a couple I loved dearly, were stuck in a toxic relationship. It got to the point where I felt like I was walking on eggshells whenever I was in their company. They broke up, and I was so relieved. But then they were talking about getting back together. I convinced them each to stay apart, and they listened to me! Sort of.

I thought I had done a great service until about a year had passed. I noticed our entire community was becoming poisonous. When I asked around, trying to get to the bottom of it, I realized what was going on. My two friends were spreading endless, vicious gossip about each other.

The split had not made their relationship less toxic. The only thing that had changed was that they were not speaking to each other. Instead, they were talking to everyone else. And everyone else was taking sides. Instead of two people stuck in a toxic relationship, a whole community was now stuck in a toxic relationship.

I should never have encouraged them to stay apart. If they had gotten back together, perhaps one of them would have finally looked in the mirror and said, "Maybe I'm part of the problem after all." But without ever having to face each other, and living entirely in a world of gossip, they doubled down on casting blame.

Even though I stopped them from getting back together in a physical sense, emotionally and spiritually I only stabilized the worst parts of their relationship. I should have stayed out of it.

Experiences like the one described above taught me to stop letting boyfriends and girlfriends vent to me about their relationships. If I let someone vent, then they might feel better. But they released some of the stress from their relationship, and now I'm stuck with it. Since I've taken on some of the stress that should be between them and their partner, it's no longer necessary for them to change their behavior. Now, whenever things get bad, they know they can unload their stress on me.

I've also stopped trying to bring people closer together. It never works, because I have to connect with each of them directly in my attempt to get them to connect. But now they don't have to connect with each other since they can just connect with me. And if they are distant because of a conflict, they might try to get me to take sides on top of using me to avoid talking to each other.

Triangles Don't Just Involve People

This is where the concept of triangles gets interesting. The triangles concept doesn't apply only to you and two other people. It also applies to you, another person, and any issue, problem, idea, value, goal, or belief.

Imagine a triangle whose three points include you, a friend, and an issue. You are responsible for your direct relationship to your friend. You are also responsible for your relationship to the issue. But if you try to control your friend's relationship to the issue, you will only stabilize that relationship's worst aspects.

An example is addiction. Almost everyone I know is stabilizing someone's relationship with an addiction. Whenever you try to control someone's relationship to whatever they are addicted to, you take some responsibility for their actions. That means they have less responsibility. They are more likely to continue their habit—except that, of course, they will go to great lengths to hide the habit from you.

The more you nag, intervene, badger, or punish, the better they will get at hiding it from you. Meanwhile, you take on the stress of their addiction. This means they have less stress. Their addiction has stabilized, and their unhealthy relationship to their addiction has strengthened.

Will reverse psychology work? Can you stop someone from drinking by encouraging them to drink? No, that won't work. Aside from the fact that they probably know what you are up to, the issue is that you are still taking responsibility for their drinking. Even if they fall for your reverse psychology ploy, they'll just take it as encouragement and as an excuse to avoid taking accountability for their own behavior.

Now, you can still define your own relationship to someone else's addiction. That side of the triangle directly involves you. You can say, as I've had to say to many addicts, "I won't hang out with you when you drink." or "I won't listen to the phone messages you leave me when you are drunk." Those healthy boundaries might change the addict's relationship to their own addiction because the whole triangle may be destabilized. But be advised that the nature of the change is unpredictable. It might not seem to be for the better, especially at first.

Triangles apply to all sorts of situations, from the serious to the trivial. They apply to you, your boss and your boss's relationship to the company's goals. If you are the boss, they apply to you, your employees, and your employee's relationship to the company's mission. Triangles apply to your relationship with a partner and any project. If you are a pastor like I am, they apply to your relationship with a congregant and the congregant's salvation. And no matter who you are, triangles apply to your relationship with anyone else and their salvation—spiritual, emotional, or financial. Triangles apply to you, your kids, and their homework. They apply to you, your spouse, and your spouse's willingness to help keep the house clean.

It doesn't matter what the issue, goal, or problem is. You cannot positively change anyone's relationship to anything else. You can only affect your own relationship to the issue, goal, or problem. If you try to control a side of the triangle that does not involve you, your efforts will blow up in your face.

And yes, these relationships can be represented by other shapes that aren't triangular. Often, in complex situations with multiple people involved, you can have various kinds of squares and octagons with many connections. The more complicated the maze of relationships, the more important it is that you focus only on relationships that directly involve you. You may even want to physically draw the shapes so you can see all the connections.

One problem to avoid, though, is just visualizing triangles for the sake of mapping them out. Don't do that! The point is not to make a picture, and certainly not to get overwhelmed by trying to figure out the complexities of family relationships that don't directly involve you. The point is to show you what you can affect and what you can't.

How to Use the Triangles Concept

A couple rented a room in my house, and their relationship had devolved into outright domestic violence. They had each called the cops at least once on the other, so identifying the "villain" was difficult.

Another tenant wanted me to evict the male, who was probably the more dangerous abuser. But if I were to kick him out and not her, then I would be trying to control their relationship. That would stabilize their relationship and its severe dysfunction.

Instead, I sat down with both of them when they were calm. I said, "This is going to be a short conversation. If I have to kick you out, I'm only going to kick both of you out—not one or the other. Do you understand?" They said they understood, and that was the end of the conversation. It lasted less than a minute.

One month later, the couple broke up and he moved out. She moved out a few months later. They did not move back in together—not at my house nor anyone else's. That's not bad for one minute of work on my part.

Notice I never tried to figure out who the villain was. I never tried to shame either of them. I stayed friends with both of them. I stayed connected to both of them. I made it clear that it's my house. I made it clear that I would kick them out if I needed to. But most important, I made it absolutely clear that I would never take sides in their conflict.

I genuinely didn't care whether or not they stayed together. So I refused to absorb any of the stress, responsibility, or anxiety from their relationship. In our three-person triangle, all the stress was placed where it belonged—on their relationship with each other. Their relationship couldn't handle that stress. It became too volatile. So they broke up, which was a big improvement for both of them.

Here's another story of domestic violence and what *not* to do.

On an internet forum, I read a post by a misguided young man who had witnessed a female friend being verbally abused by her boyfriend. So he intervened. He called the boyfriend out in front of the girlfriend. In other words, he shamed the boyfriend. The next time he saw his female friend, she had a black eye.

The young man posting this story didn't seem to understand why he shouldn't have publicly shamed the abuser. He could focus only on his belief that the abuser was a bad human being.

Let's use the triangle concept to consider better ways to approach two partners whose relationship is clearly sick. Remember that in a triangle between you and two people in a toxic relationship, the key is that the stress needs to stay on the side of the triangle where it belongs. It needs to stay with the two people who are trapped in an unhealthy situation. You cannot allow your relationship with either person to take on any of the stress, because that will only serve to stabilize the abusive relationship.

One approach is to simply be friends with both people, say positive things about them behind their backs (*never* underestimate the power of positive gossip), and make sure neither gets isolated. Know that the primary objective of any abuser is to isolate their victim. By staying friends with both parties, you make it harder for that isolation to happen. On top of all that, you make it harder for the abuser to act like you are the "bad guy" trying to steal the victim away.

You can offer the victim unconditional support, which the victim needs much more than they need you to condemn their abuser. You also avoid making the mistake of thinking you know who the "abuser" is and who the "victim" is—because maybe you don't. And if you spread good gossip about positive traits of the "abuser," you encourage them to focus on those good qualities.

Most importantly, by being positive to both people, you direct the stress of the triangle to be where it belongs—in their relationship with each other.

Guilt and Shame

If you find it surprising that you shouldn't take sides in an abusive relationship, you are not alone. Therapists often report frustration in dealing with victims because the victims feel deep guilt about leaving the relationship. The therapists think, *After everything your partner did to you, and you still feel guilty for wanting to leave?* Not only that but many victims refuse to tell their therapists about being abused because they don't want to face disapproval for staying in the abusive relationship.

I believe these reactions to guilt reflect a fundamental misunderstanding of the emotion. Guilt's purpose is to keep the family together. It's common to feel guilty for leaving, no matter how unhealthy a relationship, organization, or group is. That's why the emotion exists—to encourage you to stay.

Your emotions are genuine, but they aren't always truthful. Guilt doesn't distinguish between a healthy relationship and an unhealthy one. It just wants you to stay together.

Everyone I've known to leave an abusive environment felt guilty about leaving. And then sometimes, after leaving, people feel shame over how long they stayed. Please know that shame also has a purpose—to encourage you to follow the social norms of your family or organization and to respect the power structure. Shame does not distinguish between a healthy family and a sick one, between a liberating or oppressive set of rules.

The less healthy the relationship, the more guilt and shame are involved. And the more you disparage a person's relationship—or worse, their partner—the more guilt that person feels. The more you describe the relationship as unhealthy—and the more you discuss their partner's faults or misbehavior—the more guilt and shame build.

I am autistic and I've experienced guilt maybe once in my life. I've never experienced shame. So I have had great difficulty figuring out how to talk about these emotions. But I have to discuss them, because particularly in my work with women, I must recognize their importance.

I would like to suggest, though, that the fact that guilt and shame have no hold over me might permit me to perceive these emotions with clear, unbiased eyes. Guilt and shame are not always beneficial guides. In fact, they can often lead you far astray. And the issue of an unhealthy relationship, whether it's abusive or not, is a prime example.

No matter how much guilt or shame you feel over leaving or staying, there is no reason, based just on those emotions, to conclude that either you or your partner has a problem. The relationship itself has a problem. It is a problem that might not be fixable or even worth fixing. You are worth saving, but no relationship needs to be saved.

We learn how to be mature by being in groups that display emotional maturity. We pick it up, just like little kids pick up language. The same thing happens in relationships or families that are immature. We pick that up and imitate behaviors without necessarily realizing it. The longer you stay, the more ingrained unhealthy habits become.

How to Help a Friend Who Is in a Bad Relationship

I will now describe one of my most heartbreaking realizations. As far as I can tell, in every relationship I've seen that lasted six months or longer, both people had a similar level of emotional maturity. They might have been immature in different ways. One person perhaps was narcissistic and the other codependent, but they were at about the same level.

People don't leave unhealthy relationships until they start to heal, grow, and mature while their partner stagnates. In a different context, I once asked my congregation, which at the time was a group filled with folks who had experienced domestic violence and child abuse, "If someone leaves an abusive relationship, but they don't know where they are going, where will they end up?"

The entire congregation, with one voice and at the same time, responded, "In another abusive relationship!"

If you have a friend who is stuck in an abusive relationship, give them a place to go. Instead of trying to persuade them to leave, open up doors so they'll have something worth leaving for. Show them what a healthy relationship looks like by being a good friend. Find opportunities for them to grow, learn and thrive. See, that's all your direct relationship with your friend. None of it involves your trying to control your friend's relationship with another person or issue. You're focusing strictly on the sides of the triangle that directly involve you.

If your friend needs to mature, you can't grow for them. If you try to control their maturation, then you take responsibility for it, and that means they have less responsibility. They are now less likely to move forward and move on.

Obviously, all of this applies to any friend who is in an unhealthy relationship, organization, or group, even if the situation doesn't escalate to abuse. The same principles apply in any triangle you might ever find yourself stuck in. You have to refuse to try to control whatever side of the triangle doesn't include you. And that means sometimes you have to have a non-reaction—or even a positive attitude—toward conditions you don't like.

It's easier to understand how to have a non-reaction or positive attitude toward people you don't like. A person you don't like is still a human being. Even if they are immoral, abusive, or toxic. All human beings deserve some level of respect. Everyone has a story, so when you respond to someone as a fellow human being, you can always find something positive. But it's a little harder when it's an issue or a problem, especially one like an addiction in which you feel like the problem itself is stealing someone from you.

What Is a Non-Reaction?

My father was addicted to alcohol. He drank constantly. We once took a trip to the Midwest for a family wedding, and my father drank so much he landed in the hospital. His skin was yellow. Apparently, he had been sweating blood. We visited him after his breakdown, and he looked at me with puppy dog eyes.

I said to him, "Well, I hope you don't expect me to feel sorry for you." That is what I mean by a non-reaction.

See, the exact words don't matter. What matters is that I don't react to his failing health. There is a triangle here. The three points are me, him, and his drinking. If I try to control the side of the triangle that doesn't involve me—his relationship to his drinking—it only stabilizes his relationship to his own drinking.

Even feeling sorry for him is an example of trying to control his relationship to his drinking. It's still a reaction. The only way I could have a non-reaction to my father's drinking was to make clear that I wasn't going to take on any responsibility, not even emotional or empathetic.

My father sobered up. He didn't stay sober forever, but the twelve years he was sober were the best years of our relationship. And when I remember him, I remember those twelve years.

Here's another way to describe non-reaction. This one's a positive story about who my father was as a public person.

My father understood that a pastor must meet people where they are. So when he worked with gang members, he met them on the street. He didn't care how embarrassing, surprising, or even potentially dangerous it was. Anytime he drove around the neighborhood and saw a young man he knew, he pulled up to talk to him. It didn't matter to my father if the guy was selling drugs, arguing with cops, or just hanging out.

One day he saw a young man, Omar Lewis, who he knew well. Omar was hanging out with a bunch of his OGs—older gang members who got him into the business. So my father pulled up and cheerfully talked with Omar about this and that. The other gang members knew my father and just shook their heads like, "Man, you should know this isn't gonna work. Omar is one of us."

After the small talk ended, my father said, "Oh, by the way, Omar, I just want to let you know. Don't worry about it. Everything's covered. I do funerals for free, so your family will be all right after you get shot over this stuff." Then he smiled and waved at everyone before driving away.

Omar stood there in utter shock. The other gang members burst out laughing.

All right. There are several triangles here. One obvious triangle includes my father at one point, Omar at another, and the group of gang members at a third point. That might be the most important triangle in this situation, but I want to focus on the triangle that includes two people and an issue—my father, Omar, and Omar's gangbanging. Omar's gangster lifestyle was the issue everyone else was getting judgmental about, and as it turned out, they had good reason. Omar did get shot. He lived, barely.

My father acted very differently than everyone else. On the one hand, he told the truth. He told Omar his actions could get him killed. On the other hand, emotionally, he didn't react. He told him, in a warm, humorous way, that he didn't care about Omar's gangbanging.

These non-reactions were typical strategies my father used. Did they work? Well, it's not always easy to know, since everyone's story takes surprising turns.

I will never forget a particular day when I was preaching at the church my father started. It was the early morning service, poorly attended as such early services often are. I was about to read the Gospel, when who should walk in but Omar Lewis. He said he had just broken up a fight and needed to talk to someone about it. We saw him at church about once a month after that.

Here's another story about a non-reaction. I'll skip the details because what matters is not so much what I said but that I meant it.

I was doing business consulting with a woman who was getting way too involved in the gossip among her employees. It was the sort of gossip she shouldn't even have been hearing, and if she was hearing it, she shouldn't have paid attention. Like I said, the details of the gossip are irrelevant.

She messaged me about a perceived problem. After a little bit of back-and-forth, I finally wrote her the following:

"Look, I'm going to do some thousand-dollar-an-hour consulting for free here: None of this matters. The real problem is your relationship to your employees and that you participate in and encourage gossip. And I'm not telling you this because I have any hope you're going to change. I'm only telling you this so you can never say no one ever told you. I told you."

This is the sort of text you send and think, *Well, this might be the end of the consulting contract.* The important triangle here includes me, her, and her behavior. She thought the employees were the problem, but they weren't. And in any case, I can't affect her relationship to her employees. In fact, I can't even affect her relationship to the issue, which is her own behavior of engaging in relentless gossip.

I kept things between me and her, saying, "I'm only telling you this so you can never say no one ever told you." I made sure I talked to her only about my relationship to her. "*I* told *you*." But the real key is not that I used those particular words. The real key is that I meant them.

I was tired. I was going to tell the whole truth, and I didn't care if it led to the end of my contract. And I wasn't trying to change her. I was just making certain she could never say, "Why didn't you tell me?" I did tell her.

She changed. The contract continued, and the tension in her business miraculously disappeared the moment she made it clear no one was allowed to vent to her anymore about other employees.

The Opposite of a Non-Reaction

Another way to explain what a non-reaction looks like is to describe its opposite. The opposite of a non-reaction might include gossip, blame, criticism, condemnation, nagging, or complaining. All of these reactions are controlling whether the person reacting realizes it or not.

When I refer to gossip, I mean hearsay, which is repeating what someone else supposedly said when they are not there to clarify. Gossip in this context does not refer to telling a story about someone's actions. That isn't gossip. That's a fact. When it comes to hearsay, here's another fact: you can never state what someone else said. You can only state what you heard. And what you heard has more to do with you than with the person talking. When you gossip, you hope to control the relationship between the person you are gossiping with and the subject of the gossip. In the end, you only stabilize that relationship.

Blame is an attempt to project your stress onto someone else. Criticism and nagging are attempts to control someone's relationship to an issue, goal, or problem. Condemnation of someone or something is an attempt to control an entire group's relationship to that person or issue.

Even defending your opinions is usually an attempt to control someone else. You are trying to force them to see the world as you see it, or at least to accept that your understanding of the world is valid. The more vehemently you defend your beliefs, though, the more hardened your conversation partner's opposition will be. I speak here of interpersonal relationships. Of course, sometimes you must publicly defend your opinions. The goal in that case is usually to encourage your side or to change the minds of those who are undecided.

Complaining and venting, too, are controlling behaviors. Most of the time when someone vents, they are looking for an ally. They may not admit it or even realize it. This may be why so many of us react badly if, while we are venting, someone gives us advice. Advice implies that perhaps it's the person venting who has the problem. It's common for people to say, "You shouldn't give advice when someone else vents." Well, I am suggesting here that the venting itself is usually harmful, controlling behavior.

Another example of controlling behavior is when you compromise in your head before you've even had the conversation. This happens when you think you know how people will react, so you change what you really want to say, what you want to ask for, or where you want to take your stand. But this does not give people the opportunity to clearly say what *they* want to say, to ask for what *they* want, to take *their* stand.

That's a real problem, leading to situations in which absolutely no one gets what they want. This is best explained by the famous "McDonald's problem." The McDonald's problem is sort of a modern-day parable about how, in sick families, no one gets what they desire.

The McDonald's Problem

Five people decide to go out to eat. None of them wants to go to McDonald's. But that's where they end up going anyway. How does this happen? Well, the question comes up, "Where should we eat?"

Everyone responds vaguely: "I don't know. Where do you want to go?" "I'm just hungry, you know. Where would be good for you?" "I'm really not sure. I'll go wherever all of you go." Everyone is trying to be nice, so no one states their actual preference.

Bob wants to go to California Burrito, but he doesn't want to be selfish. After all, who wants to be the jerk who makes everybody else go where he wants to go? Not Bob. Besides, the group has never been to California Burrito.

Bob wants everyone to like him, so Bob thinks about where the group has gone before. He remembers that last week they went to McDonald's. Bob doesn't even like McDonald's all that much, but he wants to be nice and unselfish.

Bob says, "Well, we went to McDonald's last week."

Jerome wants a burrito right now. He's craving it. But he hasn't eaten in a while, and he's hungry. McDonald's is OK, but he doesn't love it. It wouldn't be his tenth choice, let alone his first. But he wants the group to make a decision, because he's freaking hungry.

Jerome says, "You know, McDonald's is cool. I'll eat whatever."

Now there's Jose. Jose loves California Burrito. But Jose doesn't like confrontation. He doesn't like to argue. He doesn't want to be the guy who causes dissension and unhappiness. So even though Jose loves California Burrito...

Jose says, "I guess McDonald's is fine."

Lisa hates McDonald's. She is about to suggest California Burrito, but she doesn't want to come off as too pushy. She doesn't want to be that aggressive female nobody likes. Before making suggestions, she likes to feel 100 percent sure everyone will be OK with them. She doesn't want to be seen as trying to dominate the group. Remember she hates McDonald's.

Lisa says, "Oh yeah, we all had a good time at McDonald's last week. Let's go."

Finally, we've got Alex. His all-time favorite restaurant is California Burrito. But the group is obviously settled on McDonald's. Alex prefers to be part of the group. He doesn't want to eat all alone, so he decides it's better to follow along with everyone else.

Alex says, "All right, McDonald's it is!"

Not one of the five people wants to go to McDonald's. In fact, notice that not one of them actually said they wanted to go to McDonald's. If you are in a sick family, pay attention to details like this! Every single person in this group wants to go to California Burrito. And yet, they are all going somewhere they don't want to go. If any of the five had suggested what they really wanted, all five would have agreed. But no one did that.

As a result, no one gets what they want.

Of course in real life, it's unlikely that all five people have the same preference for anything. But it doesn't change the fact that if you never state your real preferences, you'll never find out if anyone else feels the same. If you start from a position of perceived compromise, then you are trying to read other people's minds. You are trying to guess what they want instead of asking and listening. Worse, you are changing your own desires to fit a mere guess as to what other people want.

This McDonald's problem is a cute, easy example. But think about the same principle in terms of complaining, venting, and gossip. When you gossip about someone, you are not giving anyone—including the people participating in the gossip—the opportunity to say what they need to say to the person they need to say it to. The same happens with venting and complaining. None of it helps anyone get what they want. Not only does it avoid direct connection but the longer it goes on, the more it pushes people apart.

If you are part of a family—especially a work family—in which no one is abusive, but it seems the family is always stuck, think about the McDonald's problem. Sometimes there are ways to get almost everyone more of what they desire. If people get out of the habit of trying to get into each other's heads, then maybe they will start sharing and listening instead.

Don't Take Sides, Even with Your Past Self

To illustrate how to heal a family that is stuck in its own version of the McDonald's problem, I'm going to give you some of the most cliché advice ever committed to print: *Go after what you really want. Take action. Always do your best. Admit when you're wrong.* Those four statements are not innovative, but I'd like to show you how they all work together.

Admitting when I'm wrong means doing more than saying the words. It means changing course, altering my behavior. Taking action means having a strong bias toward action instead of just thinking, learning, or talking. It's much easier to get up and try a course of action if I know that when I find out I'm wrong, I'll just change direction. I'll try something else.

It's also much easier to have a bias toward action if I always do my best. This means that on a minute-by-minute basis, I always try my best. I always think my best, I always speak my best, and I always listen my best. (Maybe that advice doesn't sound so cliché now.) When I know I didn't shirk in the slightest, I don't need to wonder if I could have done better. That makes the risks of taking action more palatable.

My business associate, Curtis, knows how to run a healthy organization. I have two favorite stories about how he operates his business. They show the real reasons some firms are more successful than others.

Curtis is a financial advisor, and he became convinced that the best way to attract new clients would be to hold a golf tournament. He invited clients, encouraging them to invite friends who might turn into referrals. He paid a top-ten professional to host the event and golf with attendees. He planned so meticulously that he researched the day of the year when, historically, it had rained least often in the Seattle area.

The event seemed to be a smashing success. Everyone

enjoyed it. I think Curtis's favorite picture of himself with his staff comes from that event, where the whole group posed outside, in the sun, in front of a golf cart.

At the event, I asked him if he was pleased with the results. He said he was, and that he had gained an excellent prospect. But I knew the client referral probably would have happened with or without the event, and Curtis had spent a ton of money. Although he was smiling and happy, speaking enthusiastically and projecting positivity, I asked him a simple question: "So, are you going to do a golf event again next year?"

"No."

There's that simple word "no" again. Sometimes it's almost as if you have to say no to your past self. You have to set boundaries with who you used to be and refuse to take sides with the old you. Curtis had been so excited for this golf event. For more than a year, he researched, prepared, gushed, and raved. He had hoped an annual golf outing would revitalize his business. But he was wrong, so he admitted that fact and moved on.

Here's the second story. Some years later, Curtis became convinced he should remodel his office to turn one wing into a presentation room. He would then invite groups of clients and encourage them to invite their friends. He poured a couple hundred thousand dollars into the remodel, and later he poured his heart and soul into those presentations.

But for whatever reason, the clients weren't that interested. After a few years Curtis realized the project was never going to work. He also had no use for the space he had spent a large sum of money remodeling. So when it came time to renegotiate his rent on the office, he cut off that room. The landlord took it and added it to the neighboring office. Curtis got a lower rent, and the landlord got a more attractive space to lease out to someone else.

What about the hundreds of thousands of dollars Curtis spent on the remodel? Well, that money was spent in the past. It was gone.

I promised that my stories about Curtis would demonstrate the real reasons some firms are successful, and others aren't. Almost every small business owner I know would refuse to do what Curtis did in the end. They would have held onto that presentation room. They would have been unable to let go. They would have beaten their head against the wall trying to find some way to use the space, because they would be unwilling to face the failure of a favorite idea.

Now, if you are part of any sick family, whether a business, a relationship, or any other group, you know how infrequently anyone admits they are wrong. When I think of every sick family I've ever been in or seen, I cannot remember a single instance of someone letting go the way Curtis did of that $200,000 remodel. People too often take their past self's side, even when the conflict is with their present self.

In sick families, people cling. But remember the triangles concept. You can't force the family to change its relationship to anything or anyone else. The triangle involving you, the family itself, and any issue or person has three sides. Focus only on your direct relationships, and accept that the third side, the family's relationship to anything else, is not your responsibility or your business.

An annoying trait is present in almost every sick family once healing begins: resistance to healthy change. When you admit you're wrong, at first people will often hold it against you. When you try your best, your efforts might be dismissed or ridiculed. When you take initiative, you'll be called selfish. Do it anyway, because the first step to healing any sick family is to remove yourself from the family sickness. Stop trying to control anyone's relationship to any other person, issue, or goal, and instead focus only on your direct relationships. *Go after what you really want. Take action. Always do your best. Admit when you're wrong.* You have to do all four on an individual level, even though the rest of the family will stay stuck at first. That's how you define your direct relationship to any issue, making it easier to stop trying to control other people's relationships. This is also how you build up the fortitude to have non-reactions to the issues and behaviors you don't like—instead, you focus on what you most care about or appreciate.

Playfulness

Earlier I stated that sometimes it's necessary to have a non-reaction or even a positive attitude toward behaviors or issues you don't like. We explored a lot of details about non-reactions. But what does a positive attitude look like? In a word, it looks like playfulness.

In many situations, people will try to drag you into triangles you ought to stay out of. And in such situations, the "just say no" philosophy isn't always a great strategy. It's true that if you want to say no, that's a good enough reason to say no. But it's also true that sometimes there are much better ways of communicating "no" than outright saying "no." Playfulness and humor are often better approaches to situations in which straightforward rejection will likely lead to people shutting down.

One of my mentors was a Native American elder named Justine. She had a large family. When old age took its toll on her and she was close to her death, Justine summoned the entire family to her nursing home. She also told me and her best friend to come as well.

We all met in the nursing home's lobby. Justine wasn't there; she was in her room. She had tasked her best friend with telling the family that Justine was dying. But the family wasn't having it. Specifically, Alice, the eldest daughter, wasn't having it. At all.

Instead of this family meeting going the way Justine had intended, it turned into a meeting centered on the eldest child and her anger about the doctor's prognosis: Justine had only six months to live. (In the end, it turned out she had three.) Alice went on a long tirade about this hapless doctor, and she wanted Justine to see a new doctor.

It took some time, but the oldest son settled his sister down enough to persuade the family to go into the room together and talk to Justine. Again, the eldest daughter tried to dominate the conversation, but that was impossible in the presence of the family matriarch. Justine was not going to let Alice have her way. Justine explained that she knew she was dying, and she did not want to die in a hospital or long-term care facility. She wanted to die at home.

However, Justine didn't own a home. So she turned to her youngest daughter, Precious, and asked her if she could live with her. Before Precious responded, other family members jumped in to say that it wasn't fair to ask. But that didn't satisfy Justine. Finally, on the verge of tears, Precious answered. "This is so hard for me because I don't want to disappoint you." But Precious felt she could not have Justine living out these last days in her already overcrowded home.

Well, no one in the family supported Justine's plan for her to leave the nursing facility. But Justine still had one card left to play. She turned to me. "Lauren, what do you think about this?"

It's helpful here to know something about my history with

Justine. When she was younger, Justine was a rebel. She was a bad girl, and she loved it. Even in our church, she was a prankster, a practical joker. She loved puncturing people's self-righteousness with a well-timed quip.

So I looked at Justine, tilted my head to the side, and got a big smile on my face. "Aw, Justine. You're always tryin' to get me into somethin', aren't you?"

Everyone laughed. Justine was disappointed, but even she had to look out the window and smile. That's exactly the sort of thing she would have said all those years ago, and she knew it.

Then her eldest son said, "You know, Justine, I haven't been visiting you enough. And I know that. I'm gonna start visiting you every week. And there's enough of us in this family. We can all pick a day, and one of us could visit you every day of the week." And that was that.

Justine didn't get everything she wanted. None of us gets everything we want. But her kids and grandkids visited her so often that she was never alone. She did not die at home, though. She died at the hospital, surrounded by those she loved and who loved her.

I share this story because there's no rulebook for playfulness. It's not possible to explain all the ways to use humor, but the right attitude will help.

One way to think about this is to consider the opposite of playfulness. The most effective way to take on stress that shouldn't be yours is to be way too serious. Taking a problem seriously, getting all self-righteous about it, is a fantastic way to ensure no one else budges in their relationship to that problem.

Think about your own life and the times when someone took something too seriously. Was that effective in changing your mind or your behavior? How about nagging—did that ever work on you? Self-righteousness? When someone else forcefully defends their opinion, does that make you more likely to change yours? How do you feel when they verbally attack you?

Think about that scene in the nursing home with Justine. Can you imagine how uncomfortable everyone would have been if I had tried to be serious? I would have just inserted myself and my ego into a situation that had a few too many egos involved already. Even if I had told the truth, "Well, you know Justine, you really shouldn't be trying to drag me into your family conflicts." I mean, come on. There is a time for speaking truths like that, sure, but that moment in the nursing home facility wasn't one of them. The last thing anyone needed or wanted was for me to be serious. My playful response to Justine's serious request made it easier for her eldest son to make the suggestion we all knew needed to be made.

I've also learned that it's by appealing to that serious, almost self-righteous side of you that people try to get you to take on their stress. They ask for "advice," but they already know what they want you to say. They just want you to feel like a superior, like an elder, so they pose as a junior asking for guidance. Or they look for empathy. They give you the puppy dog eyes, so you feel guilty about not strapping their problems on your back.

So often, this is how the most codependent member ends up controlling the whole family. They provoke crisis after crisis, and everyone responds, taking on the stress the least healthy member should be carrying. As a result, the least healthy, most codependent member never has to change. They feed on everyone's empathy, making it someone else's job to fix their problem.

This is why, when you work with an unhealthy family, it's more effective to work with the healthiest member. Too often, service providers of all sorts are encouraged to do the opposite. They focus on the least healthy member, or even worse, the member who's showing the worst symptoms.

Focus on the Healthiest Member of a Family

For a family to heal, focus on the healthiest member. In some families there is a bad guy, who usually has most of the power, doesn't see the need to change, and, when confronted, acts like the victim. Their power makes it easy for them to resist change. Even worse, the more you focus on them the more power—or at least attention—you give them. It might not be possible to weaken the family's primary abuser, but the family will change when the other members become stronger and more independent. The healthier other family members are, the less harm the bad guy can do.

In families where there is no bad guy but the family is unhealthy, it's still important to focus on the healthiest member. This is partly because the healthiest member is usually over-functioning, overcompensating, and taking on way too much responsibility.

When I was renting a house with several friends, I had taken on the task of gathering everyone's rent payments for the landlord. I was over-functioning. At some point, my friends all started fighting with one another. I was older and a little more financially secure, so it seemed almost as if people expected me to play the parental role in this household.

One of the renters, Angela, threw an absolute temper tantrum one day, damaging property. The neighbors called the police, thinking it was a domestic violence situation. Everyone calmed down, but I had had enough. I thought, *If I weren't here stabilizing this unhealthy situation, she would never act like this. She does it because she thinks that no matter how badly she messes things up, I'll clean up after her.*

When the neighbors talked to me about the situation, of course they told me they thought she should move out. I knew that was the wrong way to handle this, though. If I tried to get her to move out, she would dig in her heels, blame me, and figure out some way to stay.

I did the opposite of asking her to move out. She loved gossip and often eavesdropped on people. I knew she would hear me if I talked loudly on the phone. So I called our landlord and told him I was thinking of moving out. I told him I was looking at places on the waterfront. I said I felt like I could afford a higher rent and was tired of the neighborhood.

Two days later she texted me, "My boyfriend and I are moving out. So you don't have to leave. We'll be out by the end of the month." The house calmed down immediately, and it was downright peaceful after they left. I remained good friends with everyone who had lived in the house, including Angela and her boyfriend.

I was over-functioning in this little family, and it was keeping us stuck and sick. It would be easy to make Angela out to be the villain, but truthfully, this house was just full of people who didn't have similar ideas about living together. I was keeping everything together, and that wasn't healthy for me or anyone else. I needed to take less responsibility in this situation, not more.

I was not surprised to learn, years later, that several studies have shown that children fight more when their parents are present than they do with no adult figures supervising them. They can afford to fight when an adult is there. If things get too out of hand, they know the adult will step in. It's more dangerous if only other children are present. If things escalate too much, who will be able to stop the escalation? When I read those studies, I thought about my experiences teaching kids at summer camp but also about my experience in that house.

There are a few other reasons to focus on the healthiest member of the family instead of focusing on the "bad guy." The healthiest member can change and might be willing to change, while the least healthy member is often unwilling to budge. Also, the sicker the family, the higher the likelihood of negative reactions to any healing. It is the healthiest members who are best positioned to withstand the inevitable blowback that comes with destabilization.

Also, the healthiest members are the ones most able to create positive emotional energy, which transforms the whole group. This transformation creates an environment in which everyone else has the opportunity to heal. This is so important that I devote the entirety of Chapter 7 to emotional energy.

In any sick family, the healthiest member is the one who needs to change. And the healthiest family member might be you. If you are the only one who can see what is going awry in your family, organization, or relationship, then congratulations! You are the healthiest member, so you are the one who will probably have to change. Maybe the change you need to make is to leave. Or perhaps you need to let people experience the anxiety and stress caused by their own behavior, which will in turn destabilize the family and disrupt its unhealthy patterns.

Never fear destabilizing a sick family. Unhealthy families need stability. Healthy families don't require stabilization because they organically create emotional energy, which causes people to want to participate in a positive group dynamic. The family has forward momentum, which is more attractive than stability. People in the family express their true selves and their individuality, and that spurs originality and creativity. Never let people blame you for refusing to keep a family stable. Only sick families require stabilization. Healthy families grow and thrive.

How to Start Healing Any Sick Family

OK, let's review. Anyone can start healing a sick family, even if you have no idea who the "bad guys" are or if there are any "bad guys" at all. Regardless of your position in the family or what kind of family you are dealing with, the first two steps to healing are always the same.

1. Set clear, consistent boundaries.
2. Connect with everyone directly.

Let's talk about step one: boundaries. The sicker the family, the more the boundaries need to be clear, non-negotiable, and almost extreme. For instance, you will probably have to set the following boundary around gossip: "I refuse to have a conversation about what another person said unless that person is present." In a healthy family, that boundary might be considered too extreme, but in a sick family, it may be necessary.

For a sick family, other boundaries might have to be just as strict. The key is to set boundaries that leave no room for interpretation and can be enforced without help from anybody.

Now let's talk about step two: connecting. The sicker the family, the more important it is to talk directly to whomever you are angriest with. In a sick family, it's likely that whatever everyone is worked up about never really happened—someone is just being scapegoated. If you are angry, upset, or anxious, it is quite possible you are merely channeling another family member's anger or anxiety. And everyone else is doing the same! The only way to clear this up is through direct connection.

Your direct connections and healthy boundaries will start the healing process, but they might also begin to disintegrate the family. See, that endless, passive-aggressive conflict was keeping the family together. Well, it was actually keeping the family *stuck* together. I never advise people to leave a family or a relationship, but I always tell people, "If you want to leave, that's a good enough reason to leave." Sometimes you do have to leave. Other times, it's not so much that you'll have to leave the family as it is that the family will have to leave you.

If that happens, you'll be better off. In the long run, so will everyone else.

In the sickest families, even if you stay, the healing process might split the family up. If there is a bad guy, the healing process causes that person to finally start showing symptoms. Some families cannot survive when the most powerful member becomes the scapegoat. Even if there is no bad guy, the family's history might be too poisoned. In those extreme cases, the healing process kills the dysfunctional family even while it removes the poison.

Most families, though, are not that sick. They survive the healing process and become stronger, more flexible, and more vital.

I sometimes visualize families as plumbing systems. The pipes represent the relationships between people, and those individuals are the fittings that connect the pipes together.

Imagine you have plumbing in which the pipes are connected in a way that makes no sense. The pipes are much longer than necessary because they are all twisted and jumbled. There are points where the water is supposed to flow up instead of down. So at the intersections where the pipes connect, there are stoppages, pressure, and even burst pipes.

If you straighten out some pipes so they connect sensibly, you stress out the rest of the pipes that are still twisted and jumbled. When the water flows well through the straightened pipes, it worsens the blockages and bursts at the intersections where the pipes are jumbled. The only way for the water to flow freely through the whole system is for all the pipes to get straightened out.

That's similar to what happens in a sick family when someone heals. When anyone straightens out their relationships, it places more pressure on all the rest of the relationships.

So prepare yourself for anxiety and blame. A sick family cannot get better without going through a period of intense volatility, because its members will become anxious and resentful when their relationships become stressed. Don't lose hope, and don't lose your nerve. Those negative emotional responses are temporary, and you can endure the volatility. Your healthy boundaries and direct personal connections will eventually heal your relationships and stimulate the rest of the family to heal in response.

CHAPTER 4

WHY DO SO MANY OF US SEEM TO RECREATE OUR FAMILY'S SICKNESS?

Healing is difficult, though, because we carry around our family dynamics and memories in our heads. This is how we "talk to ourselves," "take care of ourselves," and, occasionally, "lie to ourselves." Since we carry our families with us, we also carry predetermined and prejudged ideas about our relationships with others. When we meet new people, we often recreate the family trauma we are used to without even realizing what we're doing.

I TAKE DREAMS SERIOUSLY. FOR ABOUT A SIX-MONTH period, I had the most puzzling series of dreams I have ever experienced.

The dreams were about moving into a new house. In the most powerful of those dreams, I was moving into a sleek apartment. The building was tall, with big windows that opened onto a view of an open grass field and then a lake or a bay. It reminded me of my dorm at Western Washington University in Bellingham, but contemporary and upscale.

I awoke from each of these dreams confused. Why was I dreaming about moving? I love my house. Buying my house was just about the smartest thing I've ever done. During the early days of the COVID-19 pandemic, I thought for sure I would miss traveling. But I didn't—because I love where I live.

Then one night, I had a dream that was the kicker. I dreamed about wanting to move and not knowing what to do with all of my furniture and belongings that were in storage.

OK, anyone who knows me knows I own almost no material possessions. I bought my first piece of furniture a year or so after buying my house—a beanbag chair. I slept on the floor most of my life. Then I finally upgraded to sleeping on a mattress. About two years after purchasing my home, I shocked myself—I actually bought a bed.

Many people interpret dreams by looking for a metaphor. They might say, "Oh, all that stuff in storage represents emotional baggage." That's not how I interpret dreams.

My mother had lived in her same house for forty years. My earliest memory is of walking into that home when my family moved in. I figured my mother would live in that house forever. Maybe she thought the same.

Well, she didn't live in that house forever. A couple of weeks after my dream about dealing with items in storage, my mother told me she wanted to move to Bellingham, where my sister lives. She sold the old house, got rid of tons of stuff, and started a new life. She now lives in an apartment with a walk-in shower and no steps, in a building with an elevator. The apartment has a view of the water, just like the house she grew up in.

When I saw the photos of the apartment building my mother was moving into, I was shocked. I shouldn't have been.

Of course, the apartment building looked just like the building I had dreamed about.

See, there's no metaphor. Those dreams weren't about me; they were about my mother. Or to be more precise, they were my mother's dreams, not mine. As soon as she moved and sold her old house with its four decades of accumulated stuff, my dreams about moving ended.

And it wasn't just the dreams that came to an end. I used to love walking around Lake Washington. I would look out at the water and admire the houses on the shores. I also enjoyed visiting real estate websites to look at waterfront properties. I fantasized about my dream home. I almost spent a large chunk of money to buy a plot of land overlooking the lake, with the idea that some day I would build a residence there.

All of that stopped when my mother moved. Suddenly, taking walks in my own neighborhood was sufficient and made me quite happy. The fantasies about living on the waterfront were over. They were never my fantasies in the first place—they were my mother's. The house she grew up in was on Lake Washington, so she got used to viewing the waters every day. One day when she was sitting in her apartment, looking out at the bay, she said, "I guess someday I might get tired of looking at this view. But it sure hasn't happened yet."

To Thine Own Self Be True

Everyone seems to love inspirational quotes such as "Be yourself" or "Live your own life." And look, I agree with all the clichés. But I've learned that living your own life and being yourself are not nearly as simple as those quotes suggest. Even your dreams and fantasies aren't always your own, let alone your desires and goals.

I wasted years, nearly decades, desperately chasing after things I didn't want. And of course, many of those were things my parents wanted. For instance, my father always wanted to be famous. One time I snapped a black-and-white photo of him for a class I was taking in high school. It turned out beautifully because his hair had varying shades of white, gray, and black. I had also caught him at a perfect angle, with the sun shining.

The photo won a prize in a competition my teacher entered and got displayed in malls and such. My father was so happy. He told the story of that photo over and over again. And long before the "famous photo," he used to go on and on about how he could have been a model, an actor, or a football player. I must have spent hundreds of hours of my youth listening to my father talk about all the things he could have been.

In the real world, my father was a pastor. And he did some wonderful work, which people still talk about to this day. But truthfully, I think his favorite part of the job was the attention.

So what did I go and do? Well, I wasted about a decade of my life trying to be a rockstar—something I didn't even want. My father was the one who loved attention. When it came to fame and recognition, he and I were opposites. I love writing, mathematics, and working alone. My father loved to look out at a crowd and be recognized at a social function. When I was a child, I enjoyed copying the periodic table of the elements from the dictionary. My father looked at me and thought, *What am I going to do with this kid?*

And look, my father never pressured me. He never told me that he wanted me to be a rockstar, a model, an actor, or a football player. I don't recall a single instance of him trying to force those ambitions on me. He passed down his desires without realizing it. And I picked up on those desires without realizing they weren't even mine.

In addition to desires, I inherited so much more from my family of origin than I realized. It's true that your primary family is whatever group of people with whom you have the strongest emotional connection. But the family you grew up in contributes to determining the triangles you carry around in your head. Actually, the family you grew up with may very well define *all* the triangles in your head.

You carry around the family structure you are used to, so let me explain what I mean by "the triangles you carry around in your head."

Mother, Daughter...Sugar Daddy?

One of the most difficult cases I've dealt with as a pastor involved a young woman named Kiana. Although Kiana's mother had a master's degree, the family was often homeless. The mother had two older daughters, but both had gone off on their own. The mother had pursued an interesting strategy for achieving family stability. She was always looking for a sugar daddy. At the time I met the family, her sugar daddy wasn't providing quite enough to give them a steady place to live. He mostly took them on fancy vacations and gave them nice gifts.

So this is Kiana's idea of a father figure, and that's the triangle she carries around in her head. There were three points: mother, daughter, and sugar daddy.

Three or four years after we met. Kiana asked me all sorts of questions about my finances. She wanted to know how much money I made, how much cash I had in the bank, what my house was worth, details about my investments, and so on. These were some specific questions, and it sure felt like someone had taught her to ask them. I wondered who that someone could be.

The next time I saw her mother, I was picking up a bunch of Kiana's friends for an event. I stopped by the place where Kiana and her mother were staying. The mother was so excited to see me. She invited me inside for some pizza. She talked about how her daughter was looking forward to the event and said, "Kiana got all dressed up for you." What a *mess*. I could go on with more details, but there's no need.

A knee-jerk reaction might be to judge the mother, but that won't get anyone anywhere. Because even when the mother wasn't present, that mother-daughter–sugar daddy triangle was there. Her mother wasn't physically present when Kiana asked me about my finances. Even when I talked to Kiana one on one, it was as if her mother were lurking. That triangle was still there, working its dark magic.

If I were to participate in this triangle with Kiana and her mother, it would be unhealthy for everyone involved. There are a few obvious things I can do to break out of the triangle. I can refuse to play the sugar daddy role. I can avoid giving gifts and special favors. Those are basic boundaries any pastor should establish anyway. But more is going to need to happen for me to have a positive interaction with this young woman. Boundaries won't be enough, and confrontation won't do the trick.

Now the biggest mistake would be for me to think that I somehow have enough wisdom or moral stature to overcome this triangle as an individual. It would have been catastrophic had I tried to create with Kiana a two-person friendship so strong or resilient that it could weaken the triangle. If I had tried that strategy, then she would only have become convinced I was interested in her mother's hopes and plans for me.

No, what worked was to form a new triangle that didn't include the mother.

I remembered when Kiana told me about her family and her troubles with them. She had particular issues with the older male members. She resented her biological father, who was out of the picture. Her extended family was distant and judgmental, according to Kiana. I had asked Kiana if she had a simple, positive relationship with any family member. She mentioned one of her older sisters.

This sister was living on her own, making a living, and refusing to follow in her mother's footsteps. She had left home and, in a sense, had left her mother, although they stayed in touch. She never rejected her mother as a person, but she rejected her mother's way of life. She had ditched the fantasy that a man would save her.

When I thought about Kiana's older sister, it brought to mind a dancer named Alyssa, who volunteered at my church. Alyssa was a little older than Kiana, and Kiana loved Alyssa's dancing. Alyssa comes from a stable family, almost the opposite of what Kiana was used to. And just like Kiana carries her family triangle around in her head, so does Alyssa. But Alyssa's stable triangle of a father, mother, and daughter is much different than the manipulative and unequal mother-daughter–sugar daddy triangle Kiana is used to.

So instead of fighting against the triangle Kiana tried to place me in, I formed a new triangle. I deliberately started hanging out with Alyssa and Kiana together. Everything changed.

To understand why everything changed, ask yourself the following questions: *In Kiana's world, who does Alyssa represent? In the triangles Kiana carries around in her head, what role does Alyssa play?* Alyssa plays the role of the older sister whom Kiana has a positive relationship with. The sister had already left the sugar daddy triangle Kiana's mother always tried to create.

Whenever Kiana, Alyssa, and I were together, no matter how many other people were around, Kiana didn't think of me in the same role anymore. The triangle was now Kiana, Alyssa (as an older sister), and me. It didn't fit for me to be a sugar daddy, because Kiana's mother was no longer in the triangle, and I was certainly no sugar daddy for Alyssa. Since Alyssa took on the role of sister, and I wasn't Alyssa's sugar daddy, I couldn't be Kiana's sugar daddy either. What a relief!

Now, with a triangle that in Kiana's world consisted of Kiana, Alyssa (a sister figure) and me, I had to occupy a new role, one that Kiana wasn't used to. I could occupy the role of a protective, or at least neutral, father figure. In this triangle, Kiana became more distant from me and closer to Alyssa. But that was good! That needed to happen because closeness would have led to familiarity. Sometimes, seeking emotional distance is the healthy choice.

After seeing positive results from the triangle with Alyssa and Kiana, I knew I was on the right track. I found other women who made good older sister types. Kiana imitated them more and more, and she quit showing interest in any aspect of my personal or financial life. In these new triangles, Kiana's behavior changed. She stopped talking about finding a man to take care of her and instead spoke of getting a job.

Interestingly, Alyssa also grew from the new triangle. She didn't have a younger sister, and Kiana's friendship forced Alyssa to ask herself a lot of questions she never would have considered had she stayed cooped up in her comfortable family triangles.

At the time the two girls had met, Kiana had a rich, much

older, emotionally abusive boyfriend. She said she wanted to stay with him because he was taking her on vacation to Hawaii.

A year into her friendship with Alyssa, Kiana had gotten a full-time job, dumped the rich boyfriend, and was asking me questions about saving her own money. She was helping her mother make rent payments. She was also prioritizing her relationship with her real older sister, making new female friends, and not letting herself view her new friends as competition for the attention of cute boys. That last change was critical. When I first met her, Kiana was too focused on finding the right boyfriend. She often pushed away her female friends in favor of boys, and that had to change for her to get better.

I could pretend I was responsible for this change, but that would be dishonest. I could not be a good influence on Kiana because of the family triangles she carried around. Anything I would have tried would have been misinterpreted. Kiana did not need me. She needed new triangles, or she needed to recreate the one family triangle that was good for her. I can't influence someone if the position I hold in their family triangle is inherently manipulative, and neither can you. No one can.

Lessons

When we carry around our family triangles in our heads, we box people in. We put people in a little twisted compartment, and we get upset when they replicate the same behaviors as the last person we put in that same box. If you had a bad relationship with your father and you keep treating people like they are father figures, then you had better expect them to disappoint, aggravate, or frustrate you the same way your father did. It's not their fault. The relationship—the family triangle—is the issue, not the individual.

Or perhaps I have a healthy relationship with my father, so the opposite happens. I carry my healthy family triangle around in my head, put some new person in that mental triangle, and then I get disappointed when the new man can't live up to my father's memory. But whether the triangle is healthy or unhealthy, the issue here is that I'm not taking notice of the actual person in front of me.

If we get too used to the same triangles, even if they are relatively healthy, we stunt our growth and unintentionally ignore real people. We also have a hard time dealing with other people who are carrying around very different types of triangles.

Often, when confronted with someone else's triangles, we attack. Even when I am in the right (and I'm probably not), it doesn't work to attack a triangle. The person just gets defensive. Remember that in most cases, the triangle someone is carrying in their head goes back to their family of origin. If I attack that triangle, the other person will feel I'm attacking their soul, their essence. It has never even worked for me to attack my own triangles. I get defensive, even when I know, deep down, the triangle I'm carrying around is unhealthy!

What can work is forming a new triangle, because then people can play new roles. Real healing can happen because the triangle isn't stable yet. It's not old, brittle, and calcified. This is so important for those of you who are stuck in families that aren't abusive or even toxic. You're just kind of stuck. This feeling of "stuckness" is common in businesses, churches, and nonprofits. The way out isn't to attack the family or even necessarily to leave it. The way out is to form new families, new triangles, and new types of relationships. The old families don't need to go. New ones need to form.

So this is why I don't emphasize leaving your family or

relationships, although I do realize that sometimes it is necessary to leave. If you want to leave, that is a good enough reason to leave. But the question presents itself: where are you going to go? So first, try to put together some genuinely new triangles. Look to see how often you repeat the same triangles, especially those from your childhood. Try to either create new triangles, or at least focus on recreating those that you have positive memories of.

It's challenging to heal without a living, breathing example of how to get better. Most of us need a real person to serve as an example, almost as a mentor. And it's difficult to find that example if you keep boxing people into the same old triangles you've always been used to. For some of you, the person you need is right in front of you, but you don't see them because you see only your own family history reflected in others' faces.

Triangles Include Issues Too

The triangles you carry around in your head can also include relationships to issues, ideas, and problems. Maybe the best illustration is money, which is an issue almost everyone has dealt with.

It should come as no surprise that, as a financial advisor, I've spent plenty of time learning about people's triangles regarding the issue of money. Since we are talking about triangles that include an issue, maybe the most common triangle in America is one made up of two spouses and their money. Since this is such a common, complex, and emotionally thorny issue, let me share my own family history surrounding money.

I came home one day and the utilities had been cut off. There was no running water. My father said, "Oh, shit." It's the only time I remember him cursing. He ran out the door.

I guess he drove to the utilities company and paid the bill. Meanwhile, I was left wondering why everyone I knew had running water except us.

This happened a few times. And it wasn't that there was no money. My father was either so depressed or so drunk that he couldn't bring himself to pay the utility bill until he was forced to. I wasn't sure why my father was in charge of paying the bills, but my mother had had enough. She took over. The utilities stopped getting shut off, but I think she was a little bit shocked at how much credit card debt there was.

So that's one experience that has dominated my attitude toward money, but it wasn't as harmful as the stories I heard. My father had an antagonistic attitude toward rich people and the attainment of financial success. He particularly got angry when people moved up in the world, maybe because he felt (incorrectly) this challenged his belief that we all live in an unfair world where the rich oppress the poor. Or maybe he was just jealous.

In any case, he judged himself by how the community perceived him. He was obsessed with image but not success. So he was a pastor who worked with low-income people. This was fine and, in fact, admirable. He did incredible work. But... sometimes he didn't get paid. And he never got a raise in almost thirty years of pastoring. On top of that, he refused to put in any effort to raise money for his church, instead relying on institutional support from his old friends at a central office. As his credit card debt showed, he wasn't always financially responsible. He was responsible enough to get us to the end of the month, but the future was always a worrisome fog.

Needless to say, this is not the best set of stories about money. How did I react to these family stories?

I rebelled in some ways, but in other ways I submitted. I

rebelled by being absurdly financially responsible. I always paid every bill on time. Even during the years I worked for minimum wage, I saved money. I never asked my parents or anyone else for support. On the other hand, I also submitted, wasting years being terrified of success.

But whether I was rebelling or submitting, I was still carrying the triangles with me. I wasn't thinking outside the shape of what I had learned from my parents and their relationship with money. Those family stories still had all the power, setting the terms of my internal conversations about money. Rebelling didn't free me, and it didn't empower me. It just created a new sort of cage where I never wanted to spend money even when it would make me happy and I never asked for help when I needed it.

I did not set myself free from these stories through self-examination or internal change. All the thinking and introspection in the world did not help. I freed myself by forging new friendships with people who had learned very different stories about money. I became friends with people who were massively more successful than I was. I became part of social circles where the entire group had different beliefs about money.

I became a part of new families with new stories, new triangles. As these new families became more important to me, the old family stories faded. They became mere intellectual beliefs. And mere intellectual beliefs, unlike emotional habits, are judged by evidence. They are subject to creative interpretation, and even to being tossed out entirely in favor of better beliefs.

As a child and young adult, I never believed I would own a house. I never believed I would be financially independent. But I became part of new families, such as networks of professionals and entrepreneurs, who just assume everyone eventually buys a house.

My primary business associate, Curtis, always assumed I'd be successful, become financially independent, and own a house. We never discussed it. It was never explicitly laid out. He never said any of these things. His attitude, though, was so ingrained that it influenced every conversation we had. And in the new triangle with him and his attitude toward money, I became a different person, almost without realizing it. I ended up doing things I never believed I would do.

Now your story is probably different from mine. Listed below are some common stories that hold people back from having healthy attitudes about money. Do any of these sound familiar?

The man who is terrified of making more money than his father made.

The woman who won't let herself make more than her husband (or even ex-husband).

The working-class person who believes that they don't deserve a house, a retirement, or nice things in general.

The kids who grew up rich and think they deserve nice things even if they never work for them.

So many of these stories are about what a person deserves. Think about whatever money discussions you heard growing up. How often were they, in some sense, about what someone deserved? Or if they weren't financial discussions, how about conversations or arguments about gifts, big-ticket items like cars, or even how much food someone got to eat?

Intergenerational Attitudes toward Money

There is a reason I told the story about my father being too drunk to pay the utility bill. When you read that, did you think something like, *Man, I feel sorry for that guy. Depression sucks.* Or *This isn't even about money! It's a story about alcoholism.*

OK, here's the deal. Your family stories about money might not be about money either. You just don't necessarily see it that way because they are your stories. So of course they seem dominating and overwhelming, but they're not overpowering. They're weak. They're frail. They're flimsy. They're just about human beings and human failings. The family stories I wasted so much time rebelling against or submitting to were never powerful. They were just mine.

So I gave them away. I wrote about them, told them in sermons. Now they are no longer mine, and they no longer have any power.

Still, for the purposes of this book, there's more to the story of the triangle whose three points were my mother, my father, and the issue of money. Since I'm talking about inter-generational health, I want to share my mother's family story about money. So now I'm discussing my grandmother and grandfather on my mother's side.

In my mother's childhood home, most of the fights between father and mother were about one issue—money. That's not too surprising. Surveys suggest money is the number one issue married couples fight about. In my mother's case, the lesson she learned from her parents was to avoid discussions about money at all costs. She gave my father total control of the finances so they wouldn't fight over it.

It's kind of a sad case because she knew she was carrying that triangle around in her head—her mother, her father, and the issue of money. She tried to do the right thing because she didn't want to recreate those fights. Instead, she tried to hide from it, avoid it, pretend that somehow it could cease to exist. That didn't work. The triangle was still there. The problem didn't go away because she ignored it. Instead, it was an even bigger issue once she had to deal with it.

When my mother realized how badly (from her perspective) my father had managed the finances, it became a problem for the two of them. Now, I have to be careful here because I don't know what would have happened had my mother not taken over the finances. But from a bird's-eye view of the total history of my parents' marriage, it turned out they were financially fine. More than fine, in fact. They did well. So who knows? Maybe if they had communicated the whole time about money, it would never have become an issue.

My parents couldn't communicate about money because they didn't have a model of how to do that. Neither of them had a good family story of money. Without finding a new story, a new triangle, good communication was impossible.

My parents did communicate about most things, and they even argued openly about some issues. And speaking of the way we carry our triangles around in our heads, sometimes I can hear their voices when I think about the issues they discussed in front of my sister and me. What I mean is that, when I think, the thinking voice often sounds like my mother or father. I clearly hear their voices. I don't carry just my parents' stories with me. I carry their voices, too.

Few things helped me understand intergenerational health

and sickness more than breaking down what happens when I think—when I hear those different voices in my own head.

Self-Compassion

Yes, we've all got voices in our heads. That's not a joke, and I'm not talking about mental illness. We do contain multitudes, all of us. This is why we unironically say things like this:

- "I just couldn't help myself."
- "I lost control of my emotions."
- "I don't know why I keep screwing things up for myself."
- "I really surprised myself. I didn't think I had the courage to do that."
- "I don't know why I do precisely the things that I hate doing."

In these types of statements, who is "I" and who is "myself"? Consider one of the most famous statements from the Apostle, Paul: "I do not understand what I do. For what I want to do, I do not do, but what I hate, I do." Almost everyone can identify with this statement. Almost all of us, at one time or another, have refrained from doing what we really wanted to do. Instead, we did what disgusts us. We did what we hate.

When I say something like "What I hate, I do," it sure feels like this word "I" might stand for more than one thing. Well, my life got a lot easier when I admitted that there seem to be several "I's" inside my head. These are different selves that come out depending on the social situation or which family I'm engaging with. And these different selves don't always agree with one another.

Now, I have a conscious mind, which is always telling stories. My conscious mind tries to tell a story that feels consistent, one in which all the different voices bickering inside me sort of agree. On top of that, my conscious mind tries to tell the story in such a way that *it* plays the most important role in the story. My conscious mind is like a stage director who wants the story to be simple, but all the actors keep improvising. Many times the actors don't like the director all that much, and they undermine his perceived authority. Other times, the actors respond well only to certain kinds of direction.

Do you sometimes feel like trying to get all the voices in your head to agree is like trying to herd a flock of cats and kittens, some of whom are quite cute, but none of whom are necessarily going to do as you say? Do you ever feel like your conscious mind tries to cast itself as the most important part of the production, but the script is being written by someone else? And does the scriptwriter sometimes feel like a shadowy, hard-to-find character who lurks in the recesses of your mind and is only occasionally revealed in dreams?

Well, I'd say that's reality. And by the way, if you enjoy reading about science, contemporary neuroscience has plenty to say about the fact that we all have multiple selves. I'm not expert enough to pretend to understand all of it, but I know how to apply some of the knowledge.

First, one or more of your selves are scriptwriters. One is trying to be the director. The others are the actors. The actors don't always follow the script in the short run, but they tend to follow it in the long run. The directors sometimes succeed in getting the actors in line, but often succeed only in making them distraught enough to go way off script.

And here's the thing—sometimes the writer is writing a bad script for you. Sometimes the director is incompetent, abusive, or way too passive. Sometimes the actors are still reacting to trauma from years or decades ago—or even from your ancestors or close friends. So it's not simply a matter of ascertaining that you just shouldn't trust this self or that self. All of them are probably a little bit flawed.

However, all of them can be talked to. That includes the deep, subconscious scriptwriter. And maybe the more important point is that they all need to be listened to. Just like the people in your life, they want to be heard. And they want to be heard without judgment. They all need compassion.

How do you learn to listen to your warring selves? How do you learn to talk to them? How do you learn to be compassionate to yourself? Primarily, you learn by listening to others. You learn by being compassionate to others. The way you treat others, in the end, is the way you treat yourself. Or maybe it's better to say that the way you treat others is the way you treat all your different selves.

So let's take a specific issue—again, money—and explore how to show compassion for yourself. Let's say that these are the kinds of comments you've made to yourself: *Why did you buy that? My God, that cost $150, and here it is just sitting in the closet. Why are you so weak willed?*

If you were to talk to someone else that way, what would be the response? They might feel ashamed. They would probably get defensive. They could feel guilty or just go straight to anger. Those emotions would cause them to harden, making them more likely to act foolishly in the future.

Well, when you talk to yourself that way, your self also reacts negatively. So here you are, causing yourself emotional pain like guilt and anger, leading yourself to self-hatred, and it's not clear that you are even changing your behavior.

A better approach is compassion: *Help me understand.*

What was going on when I bought that? What can I learn from this? How can I do things differently next time?

The Voices in Your Head Represent Real People

Recently, I learned no one is born with a fear of spiders or snakes. We learn fear by seeing it reflected in the faces of others or hearing it in their voices. However, research has shown a genetic component. We are biased toward learning to fear spiders and snakes, and we are not biased toward learning to fear flowers or frogs. So we learn to fear snakes faster, and the fear goes deeper. But it's possible to grow up without a fear of snakes or spiders as long as you never learn it from others. And it's also possible to learn as an adult to be unafraid of spiders or snakes.

Fear isn't the only emotional response that gets passed down through the generations. Trauma and family sickness can also be passed down. We are biased to react more strongly to some types of trauma or sickness than others. Unfortunately, those biases reflect a world that human beings evolved into over the course of thousands of years, but we haven't lived in that ancient world for many generations.

You might not even be aware that trauma or sickness got passed down, and the person who passed it down to you might not be aware either. Most people don't remember when they learned to fear snakes. I don't remember how I learned to talk, either. I just kind of picked it up. In the same way, I picked up my ancestors' traumas and sicknesses. And for most of my life, it just seemed normal.

Your trauma and sickness might also feel normal...until they don't. Until perhaps you start having nightmares and can't discern their source. Until the anxiety attacks happen. Or maybe you are depressed all the time and have no idea why.

Yes, sometimes you can locate a cause in your present life or even in your genetic makeup. But other times, no matter how hard you look, you don't find a cause. When you can't find the cause, consider the possibility that it's been passed down to you, just like the fear of snakes. When I considered that possibility, I figured out what worked for me. Maybe it will work for you.

I don't know how else to phrase this: I had to turn my ghosts into ancestors. I did that first by recognizing that all of the various voices in my head represent real people. Second, I had to learn the stories behind those voices. Finally, I had to speak directly with the real people behind those voices, even if they were dead.

Here is an interesting example. I do prison ministry, and I also dance. One time when I ministered at the women's prison, they asked me to dance. I said no, but I promised I'd dance next time. Then I promptly forgot I ever made that promise. The next time I showed up at the prison, they asked me to dance. I said no and that I'd dance next time. Well, I had forgotten my promise, but they hadn't. They reminded me. One of them said, "No, Lauren, you said..." in a memorable tone of voice.

A few months later, I was deciding whether to play video games or do some work. I promised myself that if I got my work done, I could play video games the following day. When tomorrow came, I tried to make the same promise again. Then I heard that voice in my head: *No Lauren, you said...* They were the same words spoken in the same tone of voice. It was her. It was the woman from the prison.

That's how easy it is for someone else's voice to be added to the group I hear in my head when I think about things, talk to myself, or try to make decisions.

Unfortunately, not all of the voices are helpful. Many come from people who were self-sabotaging, emotionally stunted, or outright abusive. Listening to those voices held me back. However, just like real people don't like to be shunned or shamed and want mostly to be heard, the voices in my head would not tolerate my attempts to silence them.

At first, interrupting voices you don't like or, in extreme cases, shutting them down can work. I'm not opposed to that as a short-term strategy because there were times when I needed to do that. But in the long term, that approach failed for me. The more I tried to interrupt or shut down the negative voices, the more powerful and devious they became. They became less conscious but more influential. They apparently decided that if they couldn't influence me directly, they'd do it some other way.

I had to learn the stories behind the voices. I had to find out why my parents acted the way they did—and their parents, and their parents' parents. Just like I carry my mother's voice with me, she carries hers with her, and on it goes back through the generations. So I could be hearing a voice from an ancestor I never met.

I also had to learn the stories of former classmates, old musician friends, business associates, and the people who have come and gone through my church. By hearing their stories, I learned to listen to each voice in my head.

Only by listening, I found out why the voices were saying what they were saying. And only after they felt heard were the negative voices willing to pack up and leave, to be replaced by better, healthier speakers. I guess the voices needed acknowledgment. Each time I determined whose voice was speaking, I had to talk directly to that person. I talked directly to them—even if they were dead—through prayer, writing, meditation, or even dreams. I told them how I felt, no matter how awful, vulnerable, or beautiful it was. I had to draw boundaries with them.

You have to talk directly to people, even if they're dead. People think I'm being creepy, or woo-woo, or hyperbolic when I say that. No, I mean it. Your dead grandmother's voice in your head is really your dead grandmother. And if she's shaming you—even if it got passed down through your mother's shame—you've got to talk to her. Otherwise, the voice won't leave you alone.

Like real people, the voices in your head want to be heard. And just like real people, it's more productive to figure out what's behind their stories than it is to try to argue with them, silence them, or shame them.

CHAPTER 5

HOW SICKNESS AND HEALTH BECOME INTERGENERATIONAL

No matter what your intentions, whenever you do not deal with sickness in any family—and your own participation in it—you pass that sickness on to the next family you are involved in. So does every other human being you interact with. This is the process by which sickness becomes intergenerational. Many symptoms you suffer from may be coming from someone you barely remember or never even met.

NOW LET'S TALK ABOUT BOTH OF MY GRANDFATHERS. My father's father, Jack (actually, Jean-Louis, but he didn't use that name), was charismatic, suave, and handsome. Everyone liked Jack. He was also a mafia associate. He killed people.

Jack disappeared when my father was five. There are two possibilities. One is that he was going to serve serious time if he didn't flee. Jack's friends in the police department—yes, he was the sort of criminal who had allies in law enforcement—

told him they were going to have to pick him up if he didn't leave town.

The other possibility is that he had to run because he crossed the wrong mafioso. We'll never know for sure what happened.

Jack stole someone else's name and social security number. That was easy, since he never had a legitimate ID anyway. He started a new life in some town in Illinois. His family never heard from him again. We learned that he had died—long after his death—only because the woman he was staying with found some information with my grandmother's maiden name. The woman knew my grandfather was from Brooklyn and had kids, so she was able to send a letter to our family.

Jean-Louis is buried in Chicago under a false name that isn't even the right ethnicity. My father never visited his father's grave. Even when he traveled to Chicago, he was always "too busy."

I saw my father cry on a grand total of three occasions. Once was when he talked about two good friends who had been murdered, shot to death in front of their kids. The other two times, he was talking about his father.

At my grandmother's funeral, my father told a story about the time Jack locked him and his sister in a closet and then just left them there. My grandmother eventually came home from work and opened the door. My father and his sister came out of the closet.

Still, everybody liked Jack. I believe my grandmother was still in love with him until the day she died. She had numerous suitors after his death. She never married any of them.

Many people ask about Jack's parents. We know little about them. I do know his mother committed suicide by drinking

Lysol. It's one thing to commit suicide. It's entirely another to do it by consuming massive quantities of disinfectant.

If you want to understand what I mean by "intergenerational family sickness," this is it.

* * *

LeRoy, my grandfather on my mother's side, was intelligent, extraordinarily driven, and incredibly disciplined. He was the family standard-bearer—his mother's first son. He grew up in a poor preacher's household with seven siblings. They were always financially strapped. But he—he was going to succeed. Upon graduating from college and discharging his commitment to the military, he moved to Seattle and started work as a Boeing aeronautical engineer.

LeRoy loved his job and was loyal to his company. He didn't always love his impossible boss, whom he called "No-heart Newhart." He bought a house on Mercer Island, right on the shores of Lake Washington. Folks, this is rich people's territory. LeRoy and my grandmother raised several kids in that house. He was so financially prudent and worked so hard that when he retired, his income wasn't even going to drop. He was quite proud of that.

But LeRoy never got to retirement.

He never got there despite being a health fanatic. His determination and willpower were legendary. When his father had a stroke, he decided he needed to eat healthy. So he did it. He completely changed his diet. And when he realized he needed to quit smoking, he quit cold turkey. He said he craved cigarettes for another decade after quitting, but he never went back.

LeRoy was intelligent, resourceful, driven, determined, and...

And he also liked to climb mountains—alone.

Just before my second birthday, when his youngest daughter was still a teenager, LeRoy fell off The Tooth, a mountain in the Cascades, and died. He was fifty-four years old.

If LeRoy had lived one more year, his wife could have claimed his pension. But she never saw a dime of it. He died too young. And if he had lived thirty more years, his children could have reconciled with him the way they did with their mother. His grandchildren could have experienced his presence.

My mother, his oldest daughter, says it took her twenty years to get over the trauma of her father's death. I think she might be looking at the past with rose-colored glasses. I'm not certain that any of his kids ever got over his death.

Fake Healing

I'm not into this fake healing, positive-thinking stuff through which you are supposed to look back at your parents or grandparents and say, "They did their best." No, they didn't always do their best. Then again, I haven't always done my best either.

I'm not a fan of fake forgiveness either. "Well, their intentions..." LeRoy, who climbed mountains alone? Screw his intentions. And Jack, who disappeared on his family? Screw him too.

Maybe Jack was just trying to avoid prison. If so, why couldn't he serve his time like a man? Then my father could have told him in person to burn in Hell...or cry in front of him...or tell him he'd love him forever no matter what...or do whatever he would have done. The point is my father could have done it.

And even if Jack was fleeing the mafia, you know what? If he hadn't fled, at least my father could have attended his funeral.

No, I don't care about my grandfathers' intentions. I care about their stories though.

If you don't learn the stories of the ghosts that haunt you, those ghosts will control you. They will possess you. And if you want to heal, you can't just mindlessly forgive the ghosts that haunt your family. You have to express your genuine feelings.

But at some point, I had to turn my ghosts into ancestors. My grandfathers are my ancestors. I'm glad for my willpower and determination, and I'm grateful for my charisma. I'm even grateful for my ability to use violence, because sometimes the world is not such a benign place.

Ghosts and Ancestors

Like many people, I advocate living your own life. That sounds like such simple advice, but it's not.

When I became a pastor, I tried to finish the work my father started because he was fleeing his own father's memory. He rebelled by being a pastor to young, disadvantaged men who didn't have fathers in their lives. He rebelled by doing good. But dealing with Jack's legacy was easier because his influence was so obvious.

LeRoy's influence was more subtle. I once mentioned to my mother that after I had achieved financial independence, it didn't feel like a triumph. It didn't feel like anything. I was surprised. Well, no wonder—financial independence was never my dream. In fact it was never my dream to retire at all. I'm an entrepreneur. I haven't had a boss since 2004, let alone a "No-heart Newhart." I'll be thrilled if I get to work until the day I die.

For years, I've been plotting my purchase of a beautiful house on waterfront property. I've always thought a big house with a view would be the pinnacle of whatever success money can buy. But every time I visit a home that's for sale, the smells of the lakefront remind me of my grandmother. And I always find some reason to say no.

Finally—and this happened only a week before I wrote the first draft of this book—I was standing on the shores of Mercer Island, looking at the city lights across the waves. And I figured it out.

A house on the lake is not my dream. It's not even my mother's dream. It's his dream. It's my grandfather's ghost.

You can spend your whole life being possessed by a ghost and not even realize it. Thank God my mother told me about LeRoy being so proud of how high his income would be in retirement. If I hadn't heard that story, I don't know that I'd have ever figured out financial independence was not my own dream.

Jean-Louis and LeRoy are my ancestors. However, no matter how many people I minister to, no matter how much I dedicate myself to the issues of prisons and justice, and no matter how often I try to help others, it will never redeem my grandfather, Jack. It will never fix my grandfather's relationship with my father.

It will never stop my father's tears.

No matter how much money I make, no matter how much money I save, and no matter how expensive a lakefront property I can afford, it will never resurrect my grandfather LeRoy.

And it can't save my mother either.

You Have a Responsibility to Heal Family Sickness

I was trying to live not just my parents' dreams but also my grandparents' dreams...and nightmares. But I hadn't even met my paternal grandfather, and the other died when I was two years old. What would have happened had I never dealt with this family history? Well, I would have passed these dreams and nightmares—these ghosts—to someone else.

My grandparents and great-grandparents were immigrants, and most came here because they saw opportunity. In some cases, though, that was a small part of the equation. The larger part of the equation was what they were fleeing in Europe. I don't know the family stories from that far back. They've been forgotten, intentionally or unintentionally. But I know that very few people commit suicide by drinking Lysol. There has to be some history there.

I also know that my ancestors carried their family history with them, whether they told those stories or not. And that history has been passed down to me, whether I understand it or not. We carry our families around in our heads. Our ghosts and ancestors follow us. So anytime an issue arises, it could be an issue from hundreds of years ago. There is no way to guess its original source.

So I can stop blaming anyone. I can stop blaming my parents, former schoolteachers, or anyone who did me wrong. I can stop blaming their parents and grandparents too. And I can stop blaming myself. Nothing is gained by putting on a detective hat and trying to figure out who's at fault. It's not my fault, not my parents' fault, and not their parents' fault.

You too can absolutely stop blaming yourself. That leads us to a second point. You have a responsibility to deal with whatever family sickness you have participated in. It's no one's fault, so that's not worth discussing. It is your responsibility because you have the power to respond. We each have a responsibility for ending the intergenerational transmission of family sickness.

So let's talk more about how family sicknesses get handed down. I always find it easier to understand a concept if I have an example. The following are three stories about emotional abuse and a fourth about conflict. All four demonstrate how family sickness gets passed down through the generations.

Story #1: Guilt

One of my friends posted on social media a long list of things that made her feel guilty. She felt guilty for spending money on herself, for saying no to working overtime, and a host of other behaviors that should not incite guilt. She wanted to know how to overcome her feelings. I cannot answer that question, but I can give some insight as to where her guilt came from.

Abusers usually call people selfish because abusers become angry when someone sets boundaries. When an abuser says, "selfish," that merely means someone has a *self* and is taking care of it. A self always has boundaries—that's what makes it a self. To an abuser, that isn't good, because someone who sets boundaries can't be controlled.

This is why I repeat over and over again that if you want to say no, that's a good enough reason to say no. "No" is the first boundary.

An abuser becomes enraged at hearing any version of "no," and their refusal to hear "no" takes many forms: Self-righteous anger if you do not pick up the phone when they call. Accusing you of not caring about the group if you decline to participate in something. Blaming you for what goes wrong in the family because you didn't do something the abuser wanted you to do. Taking credit for what goes right and acting as if what went right happened only because everybody else did what you refused to do.

An abuser will accuse you of being selfish if you buy something for yourself, if you take time for yourself, if you don't text back fast enough, if you demand that agreements be honored, or if you stand up for yourself in any way.

But here's where it gets weird. A lot of people reading this will say, "But I have all this guilt anytime I say no to anybody. And no one has ever abused me!" That may very well be true.

The problem is that this stuff gets passed on through the generations. So if your parents were abused, they may have internalized the idea that it is selfish to say no, to set boundaries, or to take care of yourself. They pass that misconception on to you, because to them it's just normal. It's what they grew up with.

It seems like the most obvious thing in the world—people shouldn't be selfish. Except that, in my own life, I have never heard anyone who wasn't being abusive (or repeating internalized abuse) make the accusation that someone else is selfish.

Every selfish person I've ever known was just sort of tolerated. They quickly got surrounded by "yes men" and others who were using them. And the people merely using them are obviously not going to make accusations of selfishness! Truly selfish people get used by their lackeys, and as far as I can tell, they seem fine with it because they're using everyone else too. If you really are selfish, why would you care that you don't have genuine friendships?

Accusations of selfishness materialize when someone gets angry that they heard the word "no." Non-abusive people often get angry or disappointed when they hear "no," but they get over it. If you have internalized abuse, though, you won't see that. You'll just see the anger, and your mind jumps straight to guilt.

If you feel guilty every time you set boundaries or engage in basic self-care, the guilt is coming from internalized abuse. It doesn't matter if you were never abused. Internalized abuse can be passed down from generation to generation, and even in groups that are not your blood family.

Story #2: She Thinks She Attracts Only Abusive Men

"Why do I only attract abusive men?" So many women with tears in their eyes have asked me something similar. Now I can finally give a good answer...

You attract men who aren't abusive. You just don't see them. Your next abuser meets you and starts saying things like this to you:

"My ex was such a freaking psycho. She was evil. Not like you. You are cool, calm, and rational."

"Man, lately it feels like everyone is against me. Meeting you is like a breath of fresh air."

"My ex, she was just twisted. Devious. Not like you. You are obviously honest, a good woman. I've needed a good woman in my life for so long."

"They are only out for themselves, and I'm not down with it. They are a bunch of narcissists, not like you. You are caring, and you obviously pay attention to other people."

What you hear is that he's calling you smart, kind, and a good woman. That's not what I hear. I hear blame. Blame, blame, blame—it's all someone else's fault.

This also applies to men who tend to end up with abusive women, except that the way she insults her ex might be a little different. She may insult him for not being man enough, being a deadbeat, or not being financially stable. She'll talk about how he didn't give her many orgasms or criticize his self-care. In any case, regardless of gender or sexual orientation, blame and shame are the warning signs.

But it's seductive, isn't it? Here's this guy, and all he needs to turn his life around is the love of a good woman. And you can provide that, can't you? You look at yourself, and maybe you've got low self-esteem. Maybe you don't have much money, but you know you have love. You can love a man, right? So, finally, here's a guy who will appreciate you.

The problem is that abuse doesn't start with miscommunication. Abuse does not start with anger. Abuse does not start with yelling. Abuse does not even start with lies and deception. Abuse starts with blame.

When you don't do what he wants, when you try to stand up for yourself, when you dare to win an argument, he blames you. Because blame is what he does best. And if he keeps doing it, you start to think that maybe it really is your fault.

Sometimes he doesn't even blame you with words. He does it with obvious body language. He withdraws his love. He doesn't acknowledge you around his friends and associates. He gets distant if you are affectionate.

And it's all so different than when he pursued you, isn't it? When he pursued you, he pushed past your no's and maybes forcefully—sometimes by arguing, sometimes with puppy dog eyes. He just wanted to hang out. He just wanted to see if you were OK. Now, you know he wants more than that, but it feels so good, doesn't it, to believe that a man cares about you?

All right, that's enough. Here's what I want to say.

You attract men who are not abusive. You don't see them because they respect your boundaries. A man who is not abusive doesn't need to hear you say no. He can feel your body stiffen. He can see your arms cross. But because of your experience, when he flirts with you and you freeze up a little, he backs off. You think, *Oh, he's not really into me.* But he is into you. It's just that he respects you. That's why he doesn't keep pushing.

Maybe he gets up the nerve to ask you on a date and you say yes. He doesn't try to manipulate, pressure, or guilt trip you into sex. You think, *Oh, he's not really into me.* Maybe. Or maybe he is into you. He just respects you.

Whether or not you have ever gotten stuck in repeated abusive relationships, I hope this section shows how someone can fall for a lover who becomes toxic. Abusive relationships usually start with love bombing. This is how the toxic pattern can be handed down unintentionally to the next generation. A parent may not even realize what they are doing, but when they get love bombed during the initial stages of a relationship, the kids pick up on that.

Perhaps the parent idolizes romantic love, particularly love at first sight. They put falling in love on a pedestal. Then that's what their kids look for when they start dating. Even if the parent never abuses their kid, they can teach their kid that an abusive relationship is normal.

Story #3: The "Apology"

Remember the story about the predatory dancer I knew? In the national street dance scene, there was a brief moment when many dancers who had committed sexual assault were getting called out publicly. It happened quickly, like a domino effect. Once one woman had the courage to step forward, other women found the same courage.

During this period, a few of the men decided to publish apologies. Unfortunately, their apologies focused primarily on their struggles with mental illness or addiction, their attempts to heal, and a wide range of other excuses. As a mentally ill person, I found these excuses pretty insulting. Depression does not cause sexual assault.

More broadly, though, these excuses were disturbing because they were fundamentally abusive by nature. Many people noticed, saying the men were playing the victim. Well, that's close to being the truth.

Abusers do not exactly play the victim. Abusers believe they really are the victim.

When I use the phrase "abuser," I refer to someone who is stuck in an abusive mindset. Anyone can become abusive, and any abusive person can stop being abusive. This is one of many reasons why you should not tag someone with the label "abuser."

I can always tell when someone is slipping into an abusive mindset. But for the purposes of this story, I'll speak from a first-person perspective: I can always tell when I am slipping into an emotionally abusive mindset. The trigger is when I become so angry about what someone did that I feel any level of retaliation is justified.

Anger comes with a burst of confidence and adrenaline, and that chemical mix is addictive. If I become addicted to anger, I need more and more of it to get that burst of energy. So I become angrier and angrier over smaller and smaller things, and it makes less and less difference whether or not those triggers happened only in my imagination.

Anger, all by itself, is just an emotion. Abuse can be thought of as the combination of entitlement and anger addiction. Entitlement is not about being spoiled or elitist. Entitlement is believing this: "My life is so hard or unfair, and *somebody* owes me!" Abuse can also be defined as the point where resentment outweighs compassion and common sense. Finally, abuse can be thought of as the consistent violation of boundaries.

In all cases, believing I am the victim causes me to be abusive.

Only by imagining that everyone else is passive, unfair, stupid, or abusive can I justify always being angry with them. Entitlement makes sense only if I can convince myself that I am a victim of circumstances, bad luck, or other people's poor behavior. When I become so angry about the disgusting, stupid, absurd things other people have done, my resentment outweighs compassion. And I cannot justify violating other people's boundaries unless I convince myself they victimized me first.

Anyone can become abusive. Just believe strongly enough that you are a victim and that your desire for revenge is justified. It's especially easy to become abusive if you are in close proximity to an abuser. In much the same way, it's easier to become addicted to a drug if you always hang out with someone who is already addicted.

This is why many abusive relationships eventually evolve into relationships in which both people are abusive. This is why, for so many of us, the only way to deal with an abusive environment is to leave. When everyone around you gets high on anger, it's hard to be the only sober one.

What does this have to do with apologies? If someone says "sorry" but still talks about being a victim, they are stuck in an abusive mindset.

Let's say my abuse is of a substance, not a person. Let's say it's meth, for example. A genuine apology sounds something like this: "I know my meth use is screwing up my job and my relationship with you. It's unhealthy, and I won't use it anymore."

If I'm genuinely apologizing, there are three key elements: I should (1) say specifically what I've done, (2) say that it's wrong, and (3) say I won't do it again. The longer an apology is, the less likely it is sincere. And vague apologies are always worthless. When someone won't clearly and specifically state what they did wrong, it's because they are trying to leave wiggle room to do it again.

Here's an example of a non-apology. "I know I'm a total loser, and I drink too much. But my job has been wearing me down, and I can't handle it when I come home and you—" I won't keep going. That isn't an apology. When he says, "I'm a loser," that's a passive-aggressive way of attacking you. He's implying that you think he's a loser. Even if he doesn't realize that, he's still playing the blame game. He's temporarily blaming himself, but the blame will eventually land on you. When he blames his job or how you act when he comes home, he's not apologizing.

Remember there is a difference between fault and responsibility. If she only hurts you when she drinks, maybe the alcohol is at fault. Brain chemistry matters. But if the alcohol is at fault, then that makes it her responsibility to not drink around you—if at all! She is still 100 percent responsible for hurting you. And it is 100 percent her responsibility to make certain she doesn't hurt you again.

Say she threatened you will never see your kids again. An apology would sound something like this: "I should not have used the kids as a threat against you. That was wrong, and I'm sorry. I won't do it again." However, if she brings up all the ways you're a deadbeat or loser, or claims you don't pay enough attention to her or that you're a failure as a father, she's continuing to be abusive. Her so-called apology is just one more manipulative trick.

Final example—he hit you. If he talks about how you push his buttons or claims he wants only the best for you so he can't understand why you don't change the behaviors that make him angry—he's going to hit you again. If he blames it on his PTSD, his depression, his mom, his traumas, or how "everyone is against me"—he still believes he's the victim. He's stuck, and it's not your job to get him unstuck.

Only accept an apology if the person takes full responsibility for the consequences of their actions. Intentions, feelings, addictions, mental illnesses, beliefs, and past trauma do not absolve anyone of responsibility.

Even a genuine apology doesn't mean the behavior will change. Addictions take work to overcome. But a real apology means there's hope. A fake apology is just more emotional abuse.

If someone is brought up in a home where fake apologies are common, the sickness gets handed down. The kid growing up may very well come to think fake apologies are normal and appropriate. They will apologize that way, even though they aren't abusive! Their kids will then experience fake apologies as normal. As a result, those kids will end up associating with people who offer fake apologies. In other words, the kids will end up with abusers.

Someone who witnesses their parents being abusive but

who avoids becoming abusive themselves can still end up teaching their own children to seek out abusive mates. And they won't even realize they're doing it.

Story #4: The Snickers Bar

Now let's take a moment to talk about what abuse is not. This is a story about conflict. Conflict is not abuse, and even some harmful behaviors are not necessarily abuse. I will use one of my own harmful behaviors as an example: pettiness, as in getting angry over minor issues.

I was riding in the car with a woman I greatly admire. In fact, she is one of my heroes. It was early morning, and she took out her breakfast. "A Snickers bar?!" I blurted out in shock and amazement. I was angry and disappointed.

Her posture changed. It looked like the wind had been knocked out of her. Like anyone who gets attacked, she defended herself. "Yeah, of course." As we drove, she kept going back to the incident in different ways. She mentioned that in Seattle, a lot of people eat healthy, and she talked frequently about her eating habits.

The comment hurt, and I could tell. My pettiness poisoned our interaction. The poison wasn't fatal, but it was poison.

Now maybe you are thinking, *But eating healthy is good.* Well, that's an important point, but there is a positive way and a harmful way to bring that up. I know my comment was harmful because her body language was that of someone who'd just absorbed a punch.

My pettiness was harmful, but not abusive. No one received blame. Expressing disappointment or disgust is one thing, and I did that when I blurted out the comment about her having a Snickers. But that expression didn't quite escalate to blame. It happened and then it was over. Even if you have an initial experience of anger or frustration, you don't have to let it escalate.

Conflict is any situation in which one person or group wants one thing and another person or group wants something contradictory. Conflict itself is not abuse. However, all human beings—me included—act differently under conditions of conflict. Until you've been in a conflict with someone, you don't know how they act in conflicts. In any stressful situation, people often regress to their least admirable or most basic behavior. Conflicts definitely fit that bill. People often revert to fight, flight, freeze, or fawn behavior. So conflict can easily look like abuse because it sometimes involves yelling, shutting down, or efforts to escape the situation.

Back to the Snickers bar—that's an example of conflict. She wants to eat a Snickers bar. I don't want her to eat a Snickers bar. Now, if that is as far as things go, then I am the one with the problem. But maybe we can use this conflict to make genuine progress.

In this case, I want her to be healthy. I feel protective of her. Those desires and feelings are good and should be encouraged. The conflict is a sign, a signal, a message. It's a sign that I need to tap into those feelings of protectiveness. Viewing my conflicts as a signal instead of a problem changes my whole perspective for the better.

Conflict is not abuse. And that's good, since conflict is inevitable. Not only is conflict inevitable, but conflict is also common in healthy families. Family members feel safe expressing their opinions and desires. In healthy families, people take risks, want the family to grow (spiritually, emotionally, economically, or in actual size), and push the family to confront potential issues before they become problems.

This means conflict happens often, and conflict is just as often handled in healthy ways.

Speaking of sickness that gets handed down, one of the worst attitudes in sick families is the idea that conflict is bad. If you grew up in a sick family, maybe it feels natural to avoid conflict at all costs. This can happen whether you grew up in a passive-aggressive family in which open conflicts were rare or in a volatile family with explosive conflicts. Either way, believing conflict should be avoided is terrible because that belief will keep you out of healthy families!

A healthy family allows everyone to openly state their beliefs, desires, and goals. Since people do not always agree and have different desires, healthy families entertain lots of conflicts. This can be a shock for anyone who grew up thinking conflict should always be avoided, that everyone should always say nice things, or that people should feel bad for dissenting. It's a particularly big shock for anyone who is used to families in which disagreement is taken as a sign of disloyalty and arguments lead to gigantic flare-ups.

Family History Is the Cause of Flare-Ups

It might seem that specific incidents cause flare-ups, but most of the time they are caused by the family history itself. They are, therefore, inevitable until the family itself changes. Here's an example from my own life.

My cousin was getting married. She is the daughter of my father's only sister. I've already introduced their father—Jack, the mafioso who fled during their childhood. My father and my aunt rarely saw each other in adulthood, and when they did it was often tense. They had dealt with their family sickness by running in two opposite directions. They both left Brooklyn, where they grew up, but he had gone to the urban West Coast while she settled in the suburban Midwest. He became a pastor who served the underprivileged, and she became a financial advisor, hoping to serve the rich. My father was a leftist, and my aunt was a staunch conservative. You get the picture.

Anyway, as we headed to the wedding, my father was drunker than I've ever seen him. And we were still in the airport! By the time we got to the wedding, my father's body had failed him. He had to be rushed to the hospital. Even after a day of recovery his skin was still yellow. He had been bleeding out of his pores.

So what caused this collapse? Did the wedding cause it? Did a stressful event cause it? Did my aunt cause it? How about my cousin? No, no, no, and no. Many people would say, "His alcoholism caused his collapse." And that's where I disagree with the normal consensus. His alcoholism was a necessary ingredient, but there was a reason he got so frighteningly drunk when visiting his sister for a major life event.

What caused my father's collapse was the entire family history which defined his relationship with his sister and had produced his alcohol addiction in the first place. When he was fifteen, my father started drinking heavily in the basement. That's when his relationship with alcohol began. So let's talk about life in my father's childhood home.

The first time I heard my father discuss his home life at length, we were at his mother's funeral. At that funeral, he told the story about the time he and his sister, ages four and six, had angered their father, who locked them in the closet for hours. As my father told this story, he and his sister took each other's hand. He talked about how when they were locked in that closet, they had held each other's hand. They cried. Finally, their mother came home and let them out of the closet.

My father had wanted that story to be about his relationship with his sister and their relationship with their mother. And that's what most people at the funeral heard. That's not what his sister heard. His sister heard a story that told the truth about their father, and she was furious with her brother for telling it.

My aunt wanted to pretend nothing negative ever happened in their home. Every time we had a conversation lasting more than half an hour, she made sure to tell me she was over her father. She didn't care about him, she said. He didn't affect her, she insisted. "Not like your dad. He just can't stop thinking about him!"

Here is an abusive family history, with two siblings fleeing that abuse in opposite directions. But after their mother's death, my father wanted to face the demon while his sister still wanted to hide.

My cousin's wedding triggered my father's collapse. Major lifecycle events like weddings, funerals, and graduations often trigger severe symptoms. But the wedding didn't cause my father's extreme drinking. Both the collapse and my father's alcoholism were symptoms of a family sickness that never healed. But if you're a kid, and you see your father there with yellow skin and blood coming out of his pores—which you've never seen until he went to a family wedding—it is easy to blame the wedding.

If you blame events, situations, or people that aren't at fault, you might spend your whole life avoiding such events, situations, and people. You might even teach your friends, your kids, and others you care about to avoid them. If you saw a lot of fighting during childhood, you can easily come to the conclusion that conflict is scary. If you saw arguments about money, you might decide that money is evil. If you experienced periods of euphoria followed by danger, which are so common in abusive households, you could be afraid of feeling good.

The worst part is that you may hand down those avoidance tactics to your kids, and they won't even know where it's coming from! They never saw the abuse. They just think the sickness is normal, so they may hand it down to their kids, your grandkids. You may very well have inherited family sickness—the one you're passing down—through similar generational channels.

CHAPTER 6

THE ROLE YOU PLAY MATTERS MORE THAN YOU THINK IT DOES

People react not to you but to your perceived role in the family. That role is a mix of the actual family role you play and whatever memories and ideas people project onto you. You also do the same to everyone around you. We live not in a world of interacting individuals but in a world of interlocking relationships—connected families.

A YOUNG MAN WHO WAS BREAKING UP WITH HIS GIRL-friend came to me and asked for advice. He had started dating her when she was a teenager. The beginning of their relationship was murky, although I'm pretty sure it was legal. I knew his girlfriend. I had helped her and her family a few times. She somewhat looked up to me. This young man had cheated on his girl and often hit on other women. But in his conversation with me, he said he was trying to let go of the relationship. He claimed she had left him and that he wanted to know how to move on.

Since he seemed so sincere, I advised him to delete all photos of her from his phone. He was stunned. He barely stuttered out a sentence; "But I have over two thousand photos of her on my phone. You want me to delete them all?"

I told him, "Yes, delete them all. Then forget about them. You want to move on, right? That's what you asked for advice on, right?"

Then he gave himself away when he said, "Even her mother is on my side and wants us to get back together." So much for trying to move on.

See, he was expecting that I would give advice on how to salvage the relationship. He could then go to his ex-girlfriend and claim I supported the idea of them getting back together. He wanted another ally to help convince this young woman, whom he had not treated well, to return to him.

When people ask for advice on how to deal with another person, they are often just looking for an ally in a conflict. And here's what I know about other people's conflicts: I should stay out of them. On top of that, my advice is my responsibility. When someone asks for advice, they might want to lessen their responsibility for the consequences of their eventual decision.

Oh, by the way, this event happened several years ago. So I can report that the young woman married a man her own age. She's happy now instead of being depressed. She and her husband bought a house together and have a child. By all accounts, they are doing well. The young man, on the other hand, still hits on teenagers, is still a financial mess, and probably still asks for advice he has no intention of following.

But here's an interesting question: Why on earth was he

asking me for advice in the first place? Why did he want me as an ally?

The Role You Play Defines You

Neither the man nor the woman in the above story had a reliable father figure in their life. So in one sense, the young man was looking to me to play that father figure role. But I am also a pastor, and as a pastor, I serve in a role that comes with a specific kind of authority. The young man already had his girlfriend's mother on his side. If he could recruit someone like me as an ally, maybe could convince his girlfriend that coming back to him was the right choice.

At first, I was offended that he would even involve me. Anyone who knows me well knows I don't even want to hear about boyfriend–girlfriend drama, let alone be asked for advice about it. But he doesn't see me for who I am. Instead, he sees my role and his own family story behind similar roles.

For a long time, it hurt my feelings to realize that other people don't see me for who I am. Some folks don't even try to see me for who I am. This bothered me right up until I realized I was doing the same to everyone else. Then I stopped being so judgmental about it.

Sometimes I'm Glad People See the Role I Play, and Not Me

Most of the time, I wish people would see me for who I am, but not always! On one particular occasion I was thrilled people didn't see me for who I was. They saw only the role I played, and thank God for that. It was the first time I presided over a funeral as a pastor.

A family I knew well asked me to perform the funeral

rites for a baby girl who died at six months of age. I knew the infant's father was in prison. I did not know much else as I prepared to go to the service. I looked at myself in the mirror and wondered, *Should I wear clerical robes? Would it be too formal? Would some people object? What should I do?*

Thankfully, I asked the family member who first contacted me—Nonie, the child's aunt. Nonie said, without hesitation, "Yes, you should wear the robes."

I arrived at the funeral parlor where the ceremony would be held. I met Nonie in the parking lot. She thanked me for being willing to do the service. She also explained that there were some complications. First, the father wasn't able to attend. He couldn't get the proper release from prison because the mother had refused to put his name on the baby's birth certificate. As a result, he had no proof he was the father.

OK. That doesn't sound good. Nevertheless, all of the father's extended family were present. The mother's extended family had also shown up. Unfortunately, the mother herself had not yet arrived.

After a brief discussion about how the service would go, I walked into the room where the wake would be held. It was divided right down the middle. On one side of the room sat the mother's family. On the other side sat the father's family. The two sides were not speaking to each other. And the baby's mother still hadn't arrived.

The funeral service was supposed to begin at two o'clock in the afternoon. It is now 2:10. Still no mother. The two sides are still not talking to each other. A member of the mother's family asks me to wait until she arrives to start. I agree.

It's now 2:30. The funeral home director walks into the room. "You must start within five minutes," she says to me loudly enough for everyone to hear.

So here I am standing in front of two opposing families at the funeral for a six-month-old girl whose father is in prison and whose mother is absent. And everyone is just looking at me, waiting for me to do...something.

I feel large beads of sweat dripping down my back, one by one. I feel each bead of sweat. A single clear thought goes through my head: *Thank God I wore these robes.*

As pastor, I knew my role. My job was not to consider anyone's opinion about who was at fault for the child's death. My job was not to consider what anyone in that room thought of me, the person who had beads of sweat dripping down his back, one by one.

Four minutes pass. I started the service. At that moment, the mother walked in. And at that moment, I was so thankful that I was not me. I was simply the pastor. My job was to serve this young girl who died before she ever had a chance to live, and to serve God. That was it.

The robes helped. They changed everyone else's attitude toward me. People looked at me as a spiritual authority, not as someone who would take sides in an unresolvable family dispute. The robes also affected my attitude toward myself. Presenting the correct external appearance makes it easier to play any role.

Now, not everyone reacts positively to a pastor's robes, but people do react. Plenty of pastors can tell stories about people avoiding them in public when seeing their vestments. At the same time and in the same places, other people immediately share their life stories when they see the robes or the collar.

I even had one friend who came to a service and photographed me with my robes. He posted it on social media and wrote, *My friends are cooler than your friends. level 50 mage!* He was using humor, being playful, but he was clearly in awe that his friend was really a pastor.

The point is that everyone views me as some combination of their history with clergy, their current position in a church, or their history with father figures. Even something as simple as wearing clerical robes triggers all that history, much of which is intergenerational.

I Do the Same Thing to Everyone Else

My grandmother on my mother's side had five children and several grandchildren. Three of her daughters had kids at about the same time, and those kids were the same gender. So I had two male cousins around my age. And then my sister had two female cousins around her age.

My poor grandmother. When it came to her grandchildren, she loved us. But she definitely kept getting our names confused. Whenever she talked to any of her grandsons, she just kind of cycled through the names until she hit the right one. It was the same with the girls.

And she did the same with her sons-in-law. She didn't immediately remember any of us extended family members as individuals. Her immediate recall of our names was based on our position in the family tree. Everyone in the same position was mentally put in the same category. So we were all just the grandsons, the sons-in-law, or the granddaughters.

I do something similar, and it's kind of weird. Two young women who attended my church usually sat in the front seat of my car when I gave their group a ride somewhere. The girls were part of different social sets and had nothing else in common. They had totally different ethnicities, radically different personalities, did not look remotely similar, and their names had nothing in common phonetically. And yet I repeatedly called each of them the wrong name! I did so when thinking about them in my head, when talking to them directly, and when talking about them to other people.

Whenever I misnamed one of them while talking to others, people gave me strange looks. These two young women had nothing—*nada*, zero—in common. "Lauren, how could you possibly get those two confused?"

I guess I must have seen them both as daughter-type figures. They each played a similar role in my life, as evidenced by their desire to always be in the front seat when I gave rides to their friend groups. They had a specific position in the car, just like they had a specific position in their little social group's family tree. And I categorized them based on the role they played in my life, not based on their personalities or even their appearance.

Here's another example involving two of the four people who played the role of best friend in my life. One is my former high school classmate, Tom, who became my best friend when we were growing up. After graduating, he moved to Los Angeles, co-founded Quest Nutrition, and then built Impact Theory, a social media empire. The other best friend is a dancer, Nico, who grew up in Mexico, ended up in the Seattle area, and mostly focuses on winning dance battles.

These two men have nothing in common. Their personalities could not be more different. They are separated in age by two decades. Different ethnicities, different nationalities—I could go on. But somehow, I called them the wrong name in my head. I got emotionally confused between them when I imagined arguments in my head with either of them. I almost called Tom "Nico" once, in person!

When I was in high school, I was only just learning how to deal with my autism. Tom played a specific role as my best friend. It was almost as if he negotiated the world of social interactions for me, because I just didn't get it. Once I asked him how it was possible to figure out who was popular and who wasn't. Tom stared at me like I was a space alien. But he did answer the question, to the best of his ability.

Anyway, part of his role was to attempt to help me with my dating skills. I was still pretty hopeless, but I probably would never have dated at all in those years if not for Tom. By the time I met Nico, I could negotiate social situations. But Nico was popular with women, he was empathetic, and he was intrigued by other people's relationships. So he played a role in my life that was similar to the role Tom had played back in high school. Nico was almost like a dating counselor—my social interactions coach.

Nico and Tom have nothing else in common, but it didn't matter to me. In my brain, they somehow became the same person because they played similar roles.

Getting their names confused may be a mere quirk of my personality, but I would get emotionally confused between them. For instance, if I was having an argument with Tom, my emotional reactions to Nico got involved. That's when problems showed up.

It's not necessarily bad if I perceive the role and not the person. It's not something you should beat yourself up over, either. But we all need to notice that we do this. Most of the time, I see everyone around me as a combination of the role they play in my family, my past experiences with people who play similar roles, and my intergenerational family history with that role. We all do this to each other all the time.

New Face, Same Role

As I said, nothing is inherently wrong with seeing the role and not the person. But there are consequences.

Struggling churches, organizations, and businesses often put their hopes in a charismatic new leader who was successful elsewhere, hoping some leadership magic will turn their family around. Unfortunately, new blood rarely changes anything. Most of the time, divided churches stay divided, failing businesses keep failing, and dying organizations fail to build any momentum.

If a family is healthy, the fact that new blood rarely changes anything is great! If you join that family, especially as a leader, you are almost guaranteed to succeed. But if a family is unhealthy, it's a huge problem. In many sick families, no leader can succeed.

I remember when the pastor retired from Holy Family of Jesus, the Cambodian church that one of my churches merged with. This pastor had started the church, had been there for decades, and had never missed a single Sunday. Everyone was worried the church would fall apart, that it might disappear entirely. I had been helping the church by preaching on alternate Sundays, but I was stepping away from my role as well. So the two most familiar pastors were leaving.

So what happened? Well, not much. The former pastor's protégé stepped into the role, and a retired pastor helped out by preaching occasionally. Everything more or less continued on as before. Attendance remained largely the same until the COVID-19 pandemic hit. The church still had its potlucks, Friday night prayer groups, and traditional Khmer songs during worship. Someone else stepped into the leadership role, and the healthy family continued to move forward.

I can't even say it was a humbling experience. It was what

I expected. That congregation had made us effective pastors, not the other way around.

My father was certainly an effective pastor of the church he started. But when he retired, divisions that had always been present among church leadership became impossible to ignore. The family was divided in half, although it tried to appear united.

The division essentially devoured two pastors and drove a third into retirement. None of my father's successors could have succeeded there. The church was divided and would never unite behind any leader. After the split, both halves of the church were much healthier.

I also think about a local dance scene I participated in. This particular scene was oriented around dance battles, which often happened out on the street. I loved this scene because it had so much energy. However, I soon noticed that the family was quite unhealthy.

At the time I joined the scene, a popular dancer I'll call King was pretty much acknowledged as the leader of the scene. People listened to him when he talked, hyped him up when he danced, and allowed him to give them advice on their dancing. When he battled other dancers, he usually won.

However, as respectful as people were to him in person, they were the opposite when they talked behind his back. The criticism was endless. They picked apart every word he spoke and every move he made. They blamed him for everything that went wrong in their dance scene. But when I asked individuals to explain what he had done that was such a problem, I could never get a specific answer. The conversation usually ended with a statement that he had a big ego and everyone hated it.

Well, big egos are annoying. But leaders often demonstrate their egos, so that didn't seem to explain what was going on.

King may have been the top dog in the dance scene, but there was a contender to the throne—a dancer I'll call Jay. Soon everyone was hyping Jay up, egging him on to challenge King. It never played out because the two of them were more or less friends. But then the other dancers escalated from talking behind King's back to openly attacking him on social media. After a while, King tired of the unending blame and negativity. He pretty much left that dance scene.

For a short time after they drove off King, the dancers seemed happy. They blamed King for the scene's conflicts and said he had nearly ruined everything. After a couple of months, Jay moved into the role of the leader. But then dancers started scapegoating Jay just as they had scapegoated King. After a while, they drove Jay out of their scene too.

Then they found a new scapegoat—and another. It kept happening. It seemed every six months or so they found a new one. Their scene never got any healthier, but it kept getting smaller as the scapegoats and their closest friends were driven off. Eventually, no one wanted to be the leader. The scene even split in half at some point, but that didn't help. Most of the dancers got exhausted with the constant drama, and both halves continued to shrink.

What was strange to me was that everyone explained the history of the dance family as if it involved a series of personal conflicts. Didn't anyone notice the revolving door of leaders who'd been turned into scapegoats? It was as if the family had a mind of its own and just kept looking for a replacement for the role of leader/scapegoat.

And families seek replacements for all roles, not just leadership. When a family member leaves, either by tragedy, by choice, or because they were cut off, the family often immediately tries to find a replacement who will play the same role.

That replacement will inherit all of the family connections, expectations, and issues, whether healthy or unhealthy, that their predecessor had. The rest of the family will consciously and unconsciously try to mold the replacement's habits and behavior to fit the role.

This is one reason it's often detrimental for a family to try to heal too quickly after the loss of a member—regardless of the reason. Families need time to grieve when someone leaves. And the more serious the issues that caused the family's loss, the longer the grieving process needs to be.

Also, if the family is sick or stuck, the loss of a family member makes change possible. If the family can avoid seeking an immediate replacement, it will have to reorganize, change its structure, or maybe even do something new. Even a role that seemed unimportant, if left unfilled, may turn out to be crucial. Leaving the wound open and refusing to fall into the replacement trap makes real healing possible.

Be careful if a family treats you like a replacement. No matter how healthy you are, if you stay too long in a sick family you eventually become sick. If you are exceptional at setting boundaries, you might resist the inherited expectations for quite some time. But the unhealthy family will eventually turn on you if you don't play the role they have assigned you. On the other hand, a sick person who enters a healthy family usually either heals or gets frustrated and moves on. There is no role for the sick person in a healthy family—there's no one for them to replace. So if they aren't willing to heal, they just sort of bounce from family to family until they find one that is as sick as they are.

Despite the tendency of families to find a replacement and then let the family dynamics recreate the exact same outcomes, whenever a new leader shows up, folks get hopeful. It almost never ends well. I think we get confused because, in a new family, leadership is more important than anything. But leadership can't always change a sick family. Families that are sick often remain so, no matter what the leader does. Meanwhile, healthy families make thoroughly mediocre leaders look like geniuses.

Sometimes It's Best to Start a New Family

So what can you do if you are the leader of a family that has been sick for generations? If you are playing the role of the leader, sometimes it's best to start a new family within the old one.

I talk about this a lot when it comes to churches. I was driving a close friend from Seattle to San Francisco so that he could visit an embassy and deal with identification card issues. This is a trip of over eight hundred miles each way. He told me, "Lauren, I've never had a friend like you who went the extra mile for me." And I thought, *Buddy, I didn't go an extra mile for you. I went an extra one thousand six hundred miles for you.*

Anyway, during this long road trip, we had plenty of time to talk. And he told me, straight up, that he would never come to church at 10:00 a.m. on a Sunday morning. He wasn't necessarily opposed to going to church, but he was not going to show up on a weekend morning. My friend's attitude is common, so many churches try to change their services to attract new members. But often, when they change the Sunday morning service, the regulars become disgruntled. Few new members show up.

What tends to work better is to start something new. For example, when the church my father founded split in half, it was immediately clear to me that the remaining half didn't have enough vitality to continue for long. So I called up the dancers I knew and told them what had happened. I told them we were going to have a "dance church" the following Sunday. Now what on earth is a "dance church"? Well I didn't know, but I was sure we could come up with something.

I invited everyone I knew to attend dance church on Sunday. Everyone asked what that was. I told them they had to show up to find out.

Lo and behold, people showed up. We improvised quite a bit of the service, but everyone enjoyed it. Through trial and error, lots of improvisation, and numerous ups and downs, those experimental services turned into a well-attended, vital dance church called Fear No Evil. From the beginning, attendance was higher for Fear No Evil than it had ever been in the traditional church, even before the split.

And what happened to the remainder of the old church? Well, we struggled along for a while. But as time passed, too many pillars of that community passed away. Eventually we merged with another congregation.

The point is that the merger would have happened no matter what. But we also started something new, and it grew in ways no one expected. Because we started something new, we could focus on opportunities instead of grumbling about the old church being too stuck in its ways. The old church could enjoy its traditional services while also participating in a vital ministry.

This worked out so much better than trying to force the old congregation to change the way it did Sunday morning services.

I had a similar experience in my accountants' organization when the COVID-19 pandemic hit. At first, everyone kind of buried their heads in the sand. No one wanted to get their members sick. Then a local chapter, led entirely by a bunch of folks in their sixties and seventies, decided we needed to connect with our members. So they set up a virtual meeting—the sort of meeting the organization held in person every month pre-COVID-19. A speaker presented continuing education and led a virtual roundtable after the online meeting.

These monthly meetings had struggled to get more than a half dozen members to attend when they were held in person. For the virtual meeting, they thought maybe twenty-five folks would sign on. Instead, the meeting had one hundred attendees, which was the maximum the platform allowed.

So since that went so well, the organization continued to host monthly virtual meetings. On the fly, members of the organization formed a whole new group whose purpose was to improvise new ways to connect with our members. Member involvement went up despite the fact that we still weren't meeting in person.

This was a professional organization that had been in decline for years. The entire time I had been associated, membership declined every year. But after coming up with so many new ways to support our membership, for the first time, we saw an increase in members! No one could believe it. The organization had created positive momentum, which many of us had never experienced. And it was happening in the middle of a pandemic.

Would this have happened had we not started that new committee? I doubt it.

This sort of thing happens in business all the time. An old business, stuck in its ways, is struggling along. And the biggest mistake, if you own or lead such a business, is to focus on fixing problems. The problems will never be fixed. Focus instead on opportunities. Many businesses have been turned around, not because they fixed anything but because new operations grew to become the core of the firm. Then the old, outdated side of the business faded away.

Just like you should always focus on the healthiest members of even the sickest families, in any stuck family you should also focus on opportunities, not problems. So if you are a leader, avoid the temptation to push your best and brightest into problem-solving roles. Instead, encourage them to be part of whatever is vital and growth oriented.

Starting a New Group or Organization

Whether it is a recently formed group or an outgrowth of an older organization, leadership matters so much when a family is formed. When starting a new family, I suggest thinking about everything you do as if you are creating DNA that will be passed down from generation to generation. Codify that DNA by writing down your family's mission and deepest core principles and values. Then emphasize those principles and values every chance you get.

Also, when starting a new group, don't limit yourself to preconceived notions about who might be interested in joining. Look around for those who might be interested in embracing your group's principles and striving to promote the group's mission.

I learned an important lesson in that accountants organization during a leadership retreat after we were finally building positive momentum. We were discussing who should be invited to serve on the board of directors. At first, everyone was just kind of going around the table, talking about inviting associates they knew. Then the most experienced leader in the group spoke up. "No, I think that's all wrong," she said. "We need to put out an all-call and ask everyone in the organization. We can't just limit ourselves to contacts we're familiar with. Because then the board of directors just becomes the group of people we already know."

She was right. Our mission had been renewed, and it would have been foolish to limit ourselves to the same group of familiar leaders. New families and families going through renewal need new blood. If you keep precisely the same people around, you risk recreating the same old family dynamics.

It's even more important to seek out new members if you are recovering from a sick family or the painful breakup of an old family. Almost every day, I remind myself of the excellent quote from pastor Tim Storey: "A comeback is not a go back."

If you are part of a group recovering from a severe setback, examine whether you are really engaged in a comeback or if you are just stuck in an attempted go-back. Because look, I get it. It's so easy to remember the excitement and the momentum and to focus on the positive memories. You may want the emotional energy of the old group, the high you used to get. But you will get that only by moving forward, not by trying to recreate history.

Don't try to hold on to the old family, not even in the most limited ways. For instance, don't try to form a new mission statement by trying to salvage chunks of the old group's mission. If you cling to the past, even in small ways, you'll bring the old toxicity into the new group.

Drama Is about the Role, Not the Person

Speaking of toxicity, I used to believe conflicts were mostly over issues. If we could deal with the issue, we could deal with the conflict. And I used to believe that drama was a product of immaturity. Boy, was I wrong.

One of the strangest lessons I've had to learn is that most conflict is about the difference between a person's actual position on the family tree and where their ego thinks they ought to be. More suffering is caused by jockeying for position than by people's wrongdoing.

This lesson was driven home hard when a certain dance scene—detailed in Chapter 2—imploded. Here we had rapists and sexual predators, but the victims were more or less willing to be rational. They were even willing to forgive the perpetrators who confessed their actions.

On the other hand, people couldn't give up the competitions for status, the minor slights, and the challenges to their egos. The biggest issues were always battles for control—perceived control over younger dancers in particular. These rivalries among peers looked like sibling rivalries or wars between cousins.

I saw this in my father's old church where the most emotional conflicts were about who got to be at the top of the family tree, who took second place, and who played the role of advisor to the pastor. I saw it in an incredible business—founded by a friend and his two brilliant partners—torn apart because of a battle that seemed to be about who should get the most credit for its success. They built a billion-dollar company from scratch, and they fought over who would be seen as the father figure.

This jockeying for position is beyond frustrating. And it is often rooted in ancient family stories. People aren't just battling for the attention or status they craved in their families of origin. They are fighting leftover battles from the slights their parents received, which were based on their grandparents' fights, which descended from arguments their great-grandparents had...and on and on.

Whenever there is serious conflict and drama rears its ugly head, remember that people care far more about your position in the family than they do about you. Your part in the drama is based on the role you play, not who you are. And you can't deal with the drama by dealing with the person, just like you can't solve the conflict just by dealing with the issue.

We all act differently under conditions of conflict. Additionally, we act differently behind closed doors, and we act differently toward people depending on their position in the family tree. Everyone knows people who treat you well if you are above them in status, but they condescend if you are below them. There are also people who are kind to you if they see you as inferior to them but are threatened by you if you are their superior or elder.

It often seems as though people care most about winning, but that isn't quite right. I've made a lot of mistakes because I assumed people would be OK if they felt they were winning. Now I understand that it's not as simple as winning and losing.

People cause drama when they feel that their role is threatened. They get defensive if their position is unstable or in question. Even the most narcissistic, egotistical people in the world will mostly just stay in their own little self-centered universes as long as the family remains stable. They know who to go to for their hits of adulation and praise, and they know who they have to defer to.

But the moment someone starts to move up, everything goes haywire.

Any change in the family structure stresses out all the other relationships. That's when the conflict and the drama appear. Even people who don't tend toward egotism will act defensive and threatened when the family itself starts to change. Of course, this is a huge problem because healing can't happen without change. Healing can't happen without people's assumed roles being challenged.

So when the family starts changing, everyone gets nervous. Even those whose roles aren't threatened start to feel anxious around other family members who are becoming defensive. Defensiveness and anxiety combine to form passive aggression, and soon these emotional states infect everyone. This is how anxiety travels through the family.

So especially if you are a leader, your role is to temper the anxiety. Your job is to be the least anxious person in the room. You must refuse to react to the defensiveness, the nervousness, and the passive-aggression.

For me, that was impossible until I learned to perceive conflicts from the perspective of family roles instead of viewing them as being related to personalities or issues.

If I keep thinking people act the way they do because of who they are, then I'm going to take their actions personally. That means I'm going to participate in the defensiveness, the anxiety, and the passive aggression. And if I think we just need to resolve some issue, then I'm going to infuriate the most volatile members of the group.

I always need to remember that I can't save a family, organization, or relationship in its current form.

If a family is consumed by drama, the family is sick. Maybe someone needs to leave. Maybe that someone is me...or you. Maybe the family needs to split in half. Maybe the family needs to change so much that everyone has to reevaluate their role. This can be scary but also invigorating and exciting.

Instead of Cutting People out of Your Life, Cut out Their Roles

Here's a common meme: "Other people's perception of you is a reflection of them."

I want to finish out this chapter by explaining why I don't agree with this meme.

Other people's perception of you is their perception of the role you play in their family tree. They are not just projecting themselves onto you.

If someone sees me as a competitor, that determines how they interpret my words and actions. Their perception is about competitors, not about me. If they see me as a friend, that determines how I'm perceived. So their perception is about friends in general, not me specifically. If someone perceives me as a father figure, then I inherit all the positive and negative attitudes they have toward fathers.

Can someone's perception of me change? Thankfully, yes, but only if my role in their family tree changes. I can spark that change by setting boundaries. For instance, let's say I'm dealing with a young man who sees me as a father figure. Let's say I also happen to know his father tries to manipulate and control who he chooses to date. I can change the way this young man perceives me by refusing to get involved in his girlfriend issues.

If I fudge on the boundary, what happens? Well, now I deal with all the baggage the man has with his father. I'm not prepared for that. But let's say the young man tries to recreate with me the messed-up relationship he has with his father. For example, he tries to get me to fudge my boundaries by asking for advice about his girlfriend.

If I stay firm, what will happen? Well, he may get frustrated or disappointed. On the other hand, he might give up his attempts to blur my boundaries. He may put me in a different role. In fact, he might even invent a new role for me out of thin air. At that point, our friendship has an unlimited upside.

What does it mean, though, if he won't accept my boundary? What does it mean if he keeps trying to involve me in his girlfriend issues? It means he has *tons* of baggage with his father, and there is no way I can deal with all that. See, I don't need to know someone's history to know that the more they want me to fudge a boundary, the more I must stand firm. Because if I can't even maintain the boundary, I certainly can't deal with all the baggage hiding in the closet.

Boundaries matter, but trying to cut people out of your life rarely works. The role hasn't gone anywhere. You may end up just finding a new person to play that role!

Do you have a friend who gets into a relationship, posts all about it on social media, and then deletes all the pictures after the breakup? It's like the person's ex never existed. And then, lo and behold, the next relationship is largely the same—same problems, same ups and downs, same patterns.

I once visited a friend who seemed to regularly be in conflict with people he labeled "abusive" or "narcissistic." After a catastrophe at his house involving a windstorm, some downed power lines, and a tree that blocked us from getting to his front door, we were sitting in a Chinese restaurant. He was looking through his phone contacts for friends he could ask for help. Slightly astonished, he said under his breath, "Wow. I've really cut a lot of people out of my life." I knew right then and there how our friendship would end. A few years later, with no explanation and no discernible cause, he ghosted and blocked me. I haven't spoken to him since.

And have you ever known a boss whose solution to every personnel problem is to fire someone? No matter what the issue, the response is the same—get rid of the employee. Then the replacement—no matter how qualified they are and to the boss's apparent shock—ends up having the same problems as the employee who was fired.

I've noticed that cutting people out of your life has become a trendy way to deal with conflict. However, that usually doesn't work. The most common result of cutting someone out of your life is that the exact same problems pop up again in another relationship. Faces change, but the situations don't.

If you dump your ex and never speak to them again, it's far more likely you will carry your issues from that relationship into the next. If you ice out your friends when they offend you, don't be surprised if you keep having to do it. And if you consistently end professional relationships by burning bridges, well, maybe it's not everyone else who has a problem.

In my whole life, I've only once completely cut someone out. That was an unusual situation. This person was abusive, of course, but the real story is that he lived in a small town and had set up his life in such a way that he had all the social and economic power in every interaction. All the people surrounding him were basically his lackeys. That is also the only situation I've been in where one single abusive person, all by themselves, was making an entire family sick—and it could only occur because that one person had all the power. I had to cut him out because he was used to always getting his way, and he just did not hear me when I said the word "no." I've never met anyone else quite that entitled.

So I don't typically cut people out, but I am quick to exit the role I play in someone's life once it becomes clear that role is unhealthy. Not only has this kept other people's toxicity out of my life, but leaving the role instead of the person has also revitalized many of my friendships and professional associations.

One close friend was driving me nuts because he always

wanted me to drive him places. So, gee, I just quit giving him rides. He soon found other forms of transportation, or other people gave him rides when they were going to the same destination. Now those drivers had company on their trips, and everyone was happier.

Here's another example. I am a leader in a professional organization. They wanted me to be the president-elect, but I wasn't interested. Another member of the organization wanted the job, but they were worried she wasn't ready yet. Well, that's why she was a candidate to be the president-elect, not president.

The woman who actively wanted the job turns out to be great at it. And since I'm not trying to do a job I don't want, I'm free to spend my time helping the organization in ways that I am good at. Everyone is happier.

Once you get over the fear of rejecting people, you realize that setting clear boundaries often leads to everyone being better off. No one likes to say no, and no one likes to reject someone. But this is the entire point of leaving the role you play in someone's life instead of leaving them as a person. You can stop being someone's partner without leaving her as a person. You can decline to be a friend's business associate without rejecting them as a human being.

Another thing that helps is to be clear about what role I am playing, what role I am asking the other person to play, and what baggage I have around those roles. And I always ask myself what I'm projecting onto the person.

Am I trying to be his father? Am I treating him like he's my son?

Am I trying to be her best friend? Am I thinking about the difference between what a best friend is to her and what it is to me?

Am I trying to be his son? Do I want him to be my mentor? Am I treating him like he's my mentor despite the fact that I never told him that's the role I expect him to play?

Am I trying to be her business partner? Her brother? Her mentor? Because those three roles don't necessarily mix.

Am I trying to be a lover? A spouse? If so, are there other roles I'm trying to play at the same time? Do those roles mix, or are they oil and water?

What baggage am I bringing in from past relationships to these roles with a new person? If I am trying to be his son, what emotional hang-ups do I have with my memories of my father?

In past interactions that went poorly, quite often, my baggage was the whole problem. Sure, the other person was new. But I was playing the same tired role. My habits associated with that role were screwing things up, over and over.

And of course, now I also ask the reverse. *Is she trying to cast me as her father? Does he want me to be a big brother? On an emotional level, can this business associate tell the difference between me and his past partners?*

I try to get people to tell me their stories. Someone's story tells me much more about what's going on than a bunch of talk about specific issues. It's important not just to listen but also to proactively encourage people to share their stories. In those stories you'll see your relationship's future.

And remember that people will usually treat you according to your role, not according to who you are as a person. When you are sitting in a Chinese restaurant with him, and even he is shocked at how many friends he's turned against, understand that you will receive the same treatment if you are playing the role of friend. The role matters more than the person.

I've also learned to be cautious about trying to play more than one role in someone's life. The more roles someone is expected to play, the less likely the relationship itself is to succeed.

I always get nervous when people speak so highly of power couples. I've observed that most power couples don't last. Sure, I can think of a few examples of people who made great romantic and business partners. But more often than not, trying to play multiple roles is a recipe for too much conflict.

One of the best employees I've ever known told me of her husband starting his own business. At first, he wanted her to be part of it. After a few months, she sat him down and explained, "You can have a business partner, or you can have a wife."

He made the right choice. They are still married. She is someone else's employee.

On the other hand, one of my favorite bands of all time was a divorced couple. They made brilliant art. They just didn't make a great marriage. It's always possible to leave the role you play without leaving the person.

Sometimes people want you only in a specific role. If you don't play that role, they leave you. This can happen with your blood family if you get sick of being treated like the child or grandchild, and with romantic partners who can't stand seeing you happy with someone else. But see, if they cut you out as a human being, then they are stuck with the failed relationship's baggage, not you.

The next time you are tempted to cut someone out of your life, consider just cutting out or changing your role. You might be surprised at the results.

CHAPTER 7

EMOTIONAL ENERGY

It is almost as if our minds exist in emotional fields the way objects exist in gravitational fields. And our habitual interactions with others, our daily rituals, produce those emotional fields. Through these rituals, many of which are also intergenerational, we create the emotional energy and well-being that invigorate healthy families.

IF I HAD TO CHOOSE THE SINGLE MODERN-DAY STORY that had the most profound effect on my life, it would be a story I first read when I was twenty. I have told this story hundreds of times, in my financial planning classes and in my sermons.

The story is from a book titled *Descartes' Error: Emotion, Reason, and the Human Brain* by Antonio Damasio. The book is about the importance of emotions. The story is about a man who had none.

This man drove to a doctor's appointment in an ice storm, and he was puzzled that so many people had skidded off the road. He was confused as to why people hit the brakes when they drove over an ice patch, since everyone should know to accelerate through those patches to avoid skidding off the road.

This man with no emotions didn't feel fear. So as a result, when he hit an ice patch, he did the purely rational, Spock-like thing: he accelerated. This sounds like an advantage, no? After all, it's easy to imagine how life might be less difficult if we were never afraid.

When the meeting was over, the doctor asked the man if he wanted to schedule his next appointment for the following Tuesday or Thursday. The man went back and forth between Tuesday and Thursday for half an hour, listing all the pros and cons of each day. There was no reason to choose one day over the other. He couldn't decide. Finally, the doctor said, "We'll meet on Tuesday."

The man said, "OK," jotted down the appointment in his notebook, got up, and left.

Studies have been done on other people who lack emotions. People with this condition can't decide between a blue pen and a black pen when asked to complete a survey. They spend hours debating all the pros and cons. What is going on?

You know how when you escalate from mere anger to outright rage, the world narrows? Your vision gets smaller? That's how emotions always work. They block out information so we can make decisions, while at the same time producing the energy for making and carrying out those decisions. This blocking of information is necessary when we make small decisions that don't matter much, and also when there is no right choice.

Emotions are most valuable when we must make decisions about situations in which it is impossible to know the right choice, but we need to stick to the decision we made. For example, it's not important which side of the street we, as a society, choose to drive on. It makes no difference at all if we drive on the right-hand side, as in the United States, or the left-hand side, as in Great Britain. But we all need to drive on the same side!

Now imagine a tribe ten thousand years ago. It might not be possible to determine whether it's best to move from or stay on the current stomping grounds, but everyone will be better off if everyone makes the same decision. That's what emotions help us do.

Remember when your parents asked, "If so-and-so jumped off a cliff, would you do it too?" OK, ten thousand years ago, if you saw your friends jumping off a cliff, you had better jump too! Because whatever is chasing them is a hell of a lot scarier than that cliff. In the faraway past, we could trust our social emotions. Now it's not quite so simple.

Feelings Are Only One Part of Emotions

Before going any further, I want to address the difference between emotions and feelings. A lot of people think their emotions are their feelings, but that is not exactly true.

Feelings are merely the tail end of emotions. First, emotions move you to action through your habits. Then, later, you feel the feelings.

Before you even feel sad, you are already drinking, overworking, or overeating. Before you even feel shame, you are already self-righteous and judgmental. Before you even feel disgust or disappointment, you are already hurting your loved ones with cold shoulders and dirty looks.

If you focus on feeling better, you will never feel better. In fact, if you focus on your feelings at all you will have a hard time. Yes, your feelings matter. They are signals. No, it usually doesn't do much good to try to change feelings. Instead, it's best to change the habitual ways you deal with your emotional responses. The feelings will follow.

Our Brains Justify Our Emotional Reactions—and That's Not Always Good

Unfortunately, our brains excel at telling us we don't need to change. Again, a primary purpose of emotions is that they give us energy to make decisions and then help us stick with those choices. That's good if the family is healthy and we are going in the right direction. On the other hand, emotional stickiness keeps unhealthy families stuck together. In general, our emotions tend to resist change, even when we make poor decisions.

Now it would be nice if our intellect were to help us out here. But our brains often do the exact opposite. We tend to use our rational powers not to improve our decision-making but instead to come up with ever more elaborate justifications for the decisions we've already made. Instead of being rational, we rationalize.

This happened so many times in my own life, and the memories are painful. I'll never forget the first woman I fell in love with at first sight. I thought she was perfect. Well, it turned out she was addicted to heroin. She kept telling me she had quit. Then she'd want to see me. Then she'd start using—right in front of me. Still, I kept going back to her. My intellect rationalized what my emotions wanted to believe—that this time she had changed for good.

Oh, and then there's the second time I fell in love at first sight. Well, this perfect woman had been diagnosed with borderline personality disorder, as I learned after a few years. She never saw any reason to change her behavior, despite her diagnosis. I quit hanging out with her and the depression I was suffering from ended the next day. And yet, after a few months, I went back to her. This cycle repeated until the relationship finally ended for good. So much for love at first sight.

I used to get angry over personal insults or trivial slights. And then, since I was angry, I looked for reasons to be angry. Now, if you seek, you shall find. If you look hard enough for a reason to be angry with someone, you'll find one. And I found all sorts of reasons. Several of them I probably fabricated, and nearly all of them I blew out of proportion.

This is how people become emotionally abusive. When I let my intellect rationalize my angry emotional responses, my resentment just builds and builds. And eventually I can't control the emotional escalation anymore. My intellect, which should question my emotional responses, instead just feeds them.

Now here's an example that applies to so many folks I know and love: anxiety. Too many people believe their anxiety in the same way abusive people believe their resentment. They feel that anxiety, it upsets them, and then they seek ways to rationalize it. If you look hard enough, you can always find a reason to be afraid. You can always find a justification for your insecurities.

This is where things get strange. Apparently, when trauma is too severe, our brains have a sort of shutoff switch that clamps down on our emotional reactions. So sometimes, when truly terrible things happen, we don't feel it—at least, not at first.

When I learned about the brain's shutoff switch, it illuminated a mystery I had struggled with for years. *Why does my brain obsess over trivial slights, conflicts over insults, and embarrassments no one besides me remembers, while at the same time I forgive people who have done awful things? Why do I seem to care more about the times I've humiliated myself than I do about the times I did something wrong? And why do I sometimes have no emotional response to a tragedy while I get all worked up over a rabbit that died in my yard?* It's that shutoff switch.

I think this might be why grief from death doesn't always hit immediately. Whenever I officiate at a funeral, I deliver a short sermon on grief. I always say, "There is no instruction manual on how to grieve." Sometimes grief hits you hard right when you hear the news. Other times it seems like nothing has happened, but six months later you'll be standing on a street corner watching the wind tumble an empty pack of cigarettes. And suddenly, your world shatters.

That happened to me after two friends, Andrew and Becky, were murdered in front of their kids. I felt nothing for months. Then, while waiting at a bus stop, I remembered a hymn. I was humming it in my head. I thought, *I need to tell Andrew about this hymn the next time I see him.* And then it struck me. There would not be a next time. I would not talk to him again, not on this earth anyway. Grief hit so hard that I felt like I didn't exist, like the world was just passing by without me. The wind was blowing an empty pack of cigarettes down the street, but it seemed as if no one was observing it. I just wasn't there.

That's the delayed reaction of grief. It's a great example of why we can't always believe our emotions. Emotions sometimes blow unimportant things way out of proportion, and other times they shut down when terror or tragedy strikes.

But wait, it gets worse. If I feel very angry, my brain assumes that something *must* have caused that anger. So it goes looking for a reason. The angrier I am, the more my brain concludes that the reason *must* be important. Regardless of the emotion, that's how people get stuck in vicious emotional cycles.

Self-Sabotage

Sometimes our brains justify our emotions in ways that lead to outright self-sabotage. This is especially true when there is fear of failure or rejection. To avoid that fear we tell ourselves stories: *Oh, that wasn't really my best. I didn't really care that much. It's not what I really wanted.*

By not committing, there is a built-in excuse. We fantasize instead of taking action since fantasy is the only place where we can avoid rejection or failure.

We continue to tell ourselves stories: *Oh, the timing isn't right. I missed my chance. I just don't feel like doing it today. Things could have been different if only such-and-such happened. Oh, it's too late to respond now.* These stories allow our egos to avoid failure or embarrassment by avoiding ever trying.

But it adds up. When I look back at how I used to live, I'm amazed that I spent most of my life pursuing goals I didn't care about. Why? Partly so that if I failed, I could honestly say, "Well, I didn't care that much, so it's no big deal." Who was I trying to convince? This is a real question. Who? Which one of the many voices in my head?

Now let me continue on the subject of self-sabotage. Here's a story about a young man in high school who is about to decide which girl to ask to the prom. He is in love with one girl. The other girl he merely likes. Which girl does he ask? He probably asks the girl he merely likes, because if she says no, it won't hurt as much. Self-sabotage is the most extreme example of how we sometimes misunderstand and mismanage our emotions.

If this young man is self-sabotaging, not only will he avoid asking the girl, but he will be angry with whoever does ask her out. That's envy, but he probably won't admit to himself that he's envious. That would sting even more. Instead, he'll come up with reasons to hate that guy.

Or more likely, he'll find reasons to hate *her*. And that combination of hatred and envy may spiral out of control.

In all these cases, emotional decisions and reactions are rationalized by the intellect. Most of these examples are negative. However, the brain does the same thing with positive emotions, which is discussed in detail in the next chapter. There are ways to apply a sort of emotional jiu-jitsu to turn this tendency toward irrationality into a friendly force. But for now, let's talk about how social our emotions are. This matters quite a lot, because if our brains tend to rationalize our emotions and our emotions are primarily social, then we are far more connected than many modern folks believe.

Emotions Are More Contagious than Any Virus

This quote comes from relationship expert Steven Stosny, "Emotions are more contagious than any virus." And I'm going to use the same example Stosny uses to explain it: road rage.

Someone is angry because they had a bad day, or they are carrying resentment because their marriage is falling apart. Or they are just mad. So out of anger, they cut you off on the freeway. If you are like almost everyone, you respond with anger. And your anger rises to their level. Now maybe you don't do anything, so the transmission of the emotion ends with you. But the point is that no virus can spread from the inside of one car to the inside of another. An emotion, though, can spread that easily.

On a larger scale, so-called news programs show how contagious emotions are. Sixteen years ago I met a financial planning client who had severe anxiety about investing in US stocks and bonds. Finally I said to her, "One of the best decisions I ever made was to stop watching television." She quit watching the news, and her entire emotional state improved. She also stopped worrying about her investments. I've talked to so many friends who say their anxiety and anger were relieved the moment they stopped watching cable news programs.

And there are far more ancient methods of spreading anxiety and resentment—like false gossip. But social media in particular takes the spreading of fear and anger to a whole new level. Sometimes I think that might be the main purpose of most social media—to spread powerful, inciting emotions.

But thankfully, it's not just negative emotions that are contagious. Hope, optimism, and courage can spread like wildfire too, especially when family leaders express those emotions. On a smaller scale, people bring their energy into the room. We can all feel it.

We can even study it. There is now a ton of research on "emotional contagion," which is a fancy phrase that describes how emotions spread. Studies show that students who are randomly assigned a moderately depressed roommate tend to become more depressed. Service employees who smile actually spread some happiness. And professional athletes really do receive a boost by playing for cheering fans.

Other research suggests that it's not just the emotions that spread. Fascinating studies led by scientists Nicholas Christakis and James Fowler show that when it comes to factors such as smoking, obesity, risk perception, and happiness, we aren't just influenced by our friends and family. We are influenced by our friends' friends. In fact, we are even influenced by the friends of our friends' friends—people we may never have met or heard of. So not only do our emotions spread throughout our social networks, but the way we deal with and express those emotions also spreads, for better or for worse.

It's clear that emotions are contagious, but it's not clear how exactly we spread them. In face-to-face communication, we might catch other people's emotions by mimicking expressions or body language. In the road rage example, maybe we pick up on other drivers' emotions by projecting our own mindsets onto them. Or maybe we have a sixth sense about other people's emotional state.

By whatever mechanism, emotions can spread in a mere instant or slowly make their way through families and organizations. Prolonged exposure to someone else's emotional state will change your emotional state.

I would suggest that for all realistic intents and purposes, our social networks are entirely emotional. It might not be an exaggeration to say our brains and bodies exist in emotional fields the way objects exist in gravitational fields. Our brains think issues are important to the extent that they matter emotionally.

Emotional Energy

Here is the definition of emotional energy: *Emotional energy is represented by the feelings of confidence, elation, enthusiasm, initiative, vitality, strength, and liveliness.* When emotional energy is at its peak, you experience excitement, ecstasy, drive, and momentum.

The opposite of emotional energy is represented by boredom, disappointment and, at an extreme, depression. You know the phrase, "It fell flat?" For instance, a moviegoer might say, "I was excited during most of the film, but the ending fell flat." That feeling of falling flat is exactly what happens when you lose your emotional energy.

When you open a gift you were anticipating, only to find out it's not what you expected, that disappointment is the opposite of emotional energy. When you get worked up for a first date only to realize the person is boring, when you attend a rally and the speech gets no applause, when you have what seems like the millionth conversation about an unresolvable issue—those experiences are the opposite of emotional energy. It's that feeling of falling flat.

A wide range of experiences represent high emotional energy. Obvious examples include the elation of a winning team as they celebrate victory or the joy people express at a wedding ceremony. Other examples of high emotional energy include the absolute focus of elite competitors, the daily momentum felt by business partners of a successful startup, and the consistent feeling of confidence enjoyed by powerful people whose status is not threatened.

On the other hand, having all your emotional energy depleted always looks kind of the same. It looks like exhaustion, depression, or indifference.

Our interactions with one another cause us to have high or low levels of emotional energy. When social interactions succeed, when they go well, emotional energy builds. When social interactions fall flat, emotional energy is depleted. This is true for interactions as small as a one-on-one conversation or as big as a rock concert.

To explain, I'll start with conversations. Sometimes we get completely absorbed in conversations, and we feel lively, fascinated, and connected. Other times, conversations are just a chore.

In most Western cultures, there is an unspoken rule that conversations shouldn't have gaps, dead spaces of silence, and that people shouldn't talk over each other. So when a one-on-one conversation goes back and forth between two people who take turns speaking and listening, it builds emotional energy for both. On the other hand, conversations with long silences tend to make people feel uncomfortable or embarrassed, depleting their emotional energy. And conversations in which two people talk over each other don't build much emotional energy either.

Sometimes a conversation emotionally energizes one person while depleting another. This can happen when one person does all the talking and interrupts the other. The talker might feel energized, but the one getting interrupted feels depleted.

In a similar way, big events like concerts, political rallies, and holiday celebrations either provide almost everyone in attendance with emotional energy, or else they fall flat and lead to disappointment. Events tend to succeed when a lot of back-and-forth exchange occurs between the participants, as well as back-and-forth exchange between the participants and whoever or whatever is at the center of the event. For instance, if someone gives a speech and the audience applauds, that back-and-forth exchange builds emotional energy. At concerts, celebrities build energy by engaging with the crowd, encouraging participation, and having the crowd cheer back.

Whether it's a big event or a small conversation, the exchange creates emotional energy. In between rock concerts and quiet conversations are a whole range of other activities that either build emotional energy or fall flat—business meetings, prayer groups, hip-hop cyphers, dances, band practices, baseball games, hunting trips. In every case, the back-and-forth exchanges between participants create emotional energy.

Now, we can also try to get emotional energy from dopamine hits like video games, drugs, or sugary food. I spent way too much time during my twenties trying to get a rush from video games and sugar. But I noticed pretty early on that even online games eventually require a social element in order to keep people playing. And it's the same with using drugs or alcohol. People usually end up needing to get together in groups or else the drugs aren't enough. In fact, it's the same with food, whether the food is healthy or unhealthy. Emotional energy often builds when dining with friends, but not when eating alone.

Purely chemical energy isn't enough. We need other people. I would also argue that people gravitate to whatever situations and environments provide the most emotional energy. This would explain a lot of things that seem irrational or unhealthy. An addict may seem to be destroying their life, but if their group of fellow addicts give them the most emotional energy they can get, then they will return to that group. And they will keep returning until they find a group of friends, a new family, that can interact with them, exchange with them, and build with them the real energy they crave.

The Importance of Rituals

We all have habitual ways of interacting with other people, and these habits are little rituals. Obviously, I am not applying the word "ritual" in a religious sense. For instance, people often talk about how they have their little "morning rituals" like drinking coffee. I use the word "ritual" to mean habitual ways of interacting.

Greetings are an example. Maybe you've never thought about greetings as rituals, but I've had to. For some time I was preaching in four different settings: First, in prisons, where we shook hands. Second, for a Cambodian church, where we bowed to each other. Third, for my street dance friends, who often gave bear hugs. And fourth, for the old congregation, where we used a warm, half-handshake, half-hug greeting.

Each of these greetings is a tiny little ritual. All of us knew how the ritual would go. And the ritual was different in each setting. The role I played in the greeting ritual was also a little bit different in each setting. And I had to make sure to use the right greeting! My Cambodian friends would not have been happy had I tried to bear-hug them. It would be considered offensive or even scary.

Most conversations can be seen the same way, as small rituals. Awkward silences are avoided through small talk, which follows distinct patterns. We use interjections to keep the conversation flowing. We have hand gestures and facial expressions that serve as cues, and common questions we know to ask.

Or sometimes we don't know. Conversational rituals are different in different places and among different groups of people. Particularly among longtime friends, exclusive rituals can develop that no one else knows about. So if a new friend tries to join in the conversation, it may take them a while to learn how to go with the interactive flow.

Of course, large events like processions, religious rites, and ceremonies are rituals. But similar ritualistic habits can be seen in business meetings, bowling leagues, and card games. Any group that regularly meets develops its own little set of rituals. There is just sort of a "way things go," and everyone in the group knows what it is, even if it's never been explicitly stated.

Rituals either succeed or fail, creating emotional energy or falling flat. There are five keys to gaining emotional energy from a ritual: focus, buildup, past experience, the element of surprise, and role-playing.

1. Focus

Often a person or object is at the center of a ritual. In a conversation, the focus could be a topic, or it could be a single person holding court. In sports, the focus is the game; in concerts, it's the musicians onstage; and in political rallies, the speaker is the focus. In smaller gatherings the focus often shifts from topic to topic or from person to person.

When everyone stays focused, that builds emotional energy. When people's attention wanders, emotional energy is depleted. This may be what makes rituals so important. Without a sense of "how things go," it's difficult for most people to stay focused.

2. Buildup

How well an interaction builds momentum also matters. If a conversation never moves past small talk, if it never progresses into passionate discussion, then it's not going to create much emotional energy. On the other hand, if you reveal too much too soon, that often stuns, embarrasses, or annoys your partner. Both conversationalists need to participate in a buildup that slowly reveals more and more about each person.

Some rituals, ways we encourage each other, always happen in a good conversation—interjecting small affirmations, mimicking the speaker's body language, laughing together, and so on. These small rituals in a conversation create some emotional energy on their own. But they also chain together so that neither conversationalist has to start over again while moving to the next subject. The next subject is then approached at a higher level of emotional energy because of the previous successful conversational rituals.

The process of emotional buildup is even more obvious around big events. The buildup usually starts long before the event takes place, through marketing, advertising, and word-of-mouth. Then, when the event starts, various smaller rituals chain together into a larger experience.

I think of all the rock concerts and music festivals I've attended. Anticipation builds even as I stand in line at a venue. Then there are the opening acts, all of which engage in some sort of call-and-response exchange with the crowd. There are times when the audience sings along, times when everyone is encouraged to dance, and times when the crowd cheers wildly.

By the time the headlining act shows up on stage, waves of anticipation have already been built up. And while all those small rituals create their own emotional energy, they also chain together so that none of the acts has to start over again to recharge the concertgoers. They build on the emotional energy created by previous performers.

This chaining together of smaller rituals is apparent when I speak publicly, particularly when I deliver a sermon. It's not easy to preach to a cold crowd. No one knows what to expect, and no one knows why I'm talking. I have to start from ground zero. On the other hand, the sermons that get the best reception happen in the context of services that incorporate several rituals that precede the sermon—usually greetings, singing, scripture readings, and prayer.

Buildup also matters during the sermon itself. I was surprised to learn that during speeches, applause usually starts up microseconds before the speaker finishes delivering the lines garnering the applause. People know when to clap and cheer. They know that the time is coming. It's a ritual, a habit that has a rhythm to it. The rhythmic applause chains together so the speaker never has to hit a restart button. The previous successful exchange between speaker and audience amplifies the next exchange.

3. Past Experience

Past experience determines how much emotional energy you get out of a ritual. If you have no experience with the ritual, you might not even know how to participate. And if you have very limited experience, you might be too uncomfortable to gain much energy.

Every time I perform a funeral ceremony, I remember every other funeral I've ever officiated. Those memories influence and energize the present moment. The memories provide depth and help me to focus. They keep me feeling confident, grounded, and strong.

This is true for every ritual, even simple one-on-one conversations. Past conversations link together in memory, providing topics, substance, and emotional energy to the current conversation. When friends get together to watch college football, their past experiences on game days, their knowledge of the sport's terminology, and their history of supporting the teams contribute to how much energy they get from the gathering. So past experience matters. But at the same time...

4. Surprise

The element of surprise also matters. It's an interesting balance. On the one hand, for a ritual to succeed people need to know how things typically go. On the other hand, if there is no variation, if there are no surprises, if nothing new happens, then the ritual becomes rote and boring. People's attention wanders.

I've noticed the most emotionally charged rituals often feature a well-known buildup, but the peak of the ritual is surprising, sometimes even shocking. Other effective rituals often feature familiar ideas, props, or characters, but they get presented in a new context.

Maybe this is why professional sports offer such consistently successful rituals. People know the rules of the game and how things are supposed to go in general. You know tension and excitement are going to build as the game progresses. Yet you don't know who will win. And the more unexpected the win is, the more emotional energy the crowd conjures.

5. Role-Playing

Everyone plays a role in a ritual. A ritual produces emotional energy for you based on whether you play your role well and whether you know you played it well. Did you feel heard in the conversation? Were you respected in the business meeting? Did you perform well during the game, show, or event? If you were part of an audience, did you feel connected when you cheered, applauded, and expressed appreciation? People feel proud and confident when they can play their role, and every single role matters in a ritual, no matter how small.

This is one reason it's so hard for people to join and commit to new families. When people feel they aren't playing their role well or that their role doesn't matter, they're less likely to want to spend what little energy they have trying new things. Too many failed interactions, especially if they are consecutive, can leave a person feeling depressed and hesitant. On top of that, it's sometimes hard to learn new rituals. So people often stick with the rituals they know, even if those rituals aren't healthy or empowering. It might be easier than taking emotional risks.

Frontstage and Backstage

Sociologist Randall Collins is one of my favorite academics. He was the first author I read who discussed human interaction in terms of rituals. He talks often about "frontstage" and "backstage" performances. Frontstage rituals are those you participate in with real people. Backstage rituals are those you practice by yourself in preparation for the frontstage performances.

Speeches and presentations are perfect examples. You can practice in front of a mirror, by filming yourself, or just in your own imagination. These backstage performances help you build confidence, identify potential flaws, and fine-tune your delivery. Then, when it's time to speak publicly, you are more likely to feel like you are standing on solid ground.

You can practice any interaction, any ritual, no matter how large or small. Practice is good and often necessary. You can use backstage practice to make it easier to engage with new families, to expand your emotional world, or to find the tribe you need and deserve.

But there is a danger that you might get too used to the backstage. You might find that your comfort zone remains in that realm of fantasy, imagination, and performance in front of a mirror. Technology today makes this danger acute. It's a little bit too easy, with the echo chamber of social media and the allure of video games, to stay backstage. The brain and body need real interaction with real people.

How to Create Emotional Energy

I believe the human brain does not see the world selfishly or selflessly. It wants to act in the best interests of the tribe. Emotional energy, produced by rituals large and small, makes your brain think you are part of a vital tribe. Emotional energy spreads because emotions are contagious, so positive emotional energy just attracts more positive emotional energy. Everyone in the family benefits, especially the least healthy members—the ones most in need of revitalization and renewal.

Every family needs more emotional energy, so let's discuss how to create it. Most day-to-day rituals that create emotional energy involve laughter, telling stories, exercise, singing, or dance. I am convinced that in our modern society, people would be happier by turning to basic rituals like storytelling and dancing, which are so central to primitive cultures.

Because we are starved for the emotional energy that we could be getting from daily rituals, we have to seek more and more of it from big, gaudy events. Occasional mass gatherings are awesome, but the roles we can play in those contexts are often limited. Participants are either the center of attention or just a face in the crowd. So if something goes wrong with the person in the spotlight, the whole edifice collapses.

It's better and more sustainable to practice a multitude of small daily rituals in which you play a variety of roles. Even the way you greet a shop owner or barista is a ritual, providing some small dose of energy. When you rehash your favorite stories with your friends or kiss your partner, those are small but necessary rituals.

In our daily lives, we can create energy by making our interactions more exciting, so there is more of a buildup. We can do that, for instance, with intentional role-playing, such as wearing costumes. I've often thought that most of the people I know would be much happier and filled with more positive energy if we were to celebrate a Halloween-like holiday every few weeks.

It's also important for me to embrace whatever role I'm in at the moment and let go of the role I just played. For instance, I play a certain role in my office. But when I physically leave that office, I don't carry that role with me. That person stays in the office, along with all of my workplace concerns and cares. When I come home and interact with my housemates, I play a different role. And when I am in that role, I don't let the person I am in my office enter my home.

Knowing what role you're playing makes it easier to gain emotional energy from the rituals you are a part of. A great benefit of stepping outside your comfort zone, meeting new people, and encountering new families is that you can access more emotional energy. However, it does not cut it to just be a tourist. You have to stick around long enough to get familiar with the rituals and your role.

The key to endless emotional energy is to participate in a variety of positive, long-standing social rituals. There is no shortcut. You have to be a part of groups long enough for the rituals to become meaningful for you. You have to get to know people well enough that your greetings, conversations, and other interactions reliably create momentum. You also can't avoid taking emotional risks. You have to be willing to commit to new activities, new roles, and new rituals. Otherwise, you will eventually get stuck.

Endless Emotional Energy

One of the best books I've ever read is titled *Dancing in the Streets: A History of Collective Joy* by Barbara Ehrenreich. She writes about dance, one of my favorite subjects, in the context of ecstatic experiences.

The author studied ecstatic experiences in many cultures, including tribal settings where people danced as a group into a sort of frenzy. They were exhausted and satiated by the end of the ritual. These ecstatic dances are common in nearly all primal cultures. In fact, dance may be an essential part of human evolution. Most predators don't have great eyesight and cannot tell the difference between 150 people stomping their feet in rhythm and one giant, 300-footed monster stomping up an earthquake. We may have used dance to survive for thousands of years, using our sense of rhythm to fool predators into thinking we were giant beasts.

Anyway, regardless of the original evolutionary value of dance, our ancestral societies all participated in rituals in which people danced to the point of ecstasy. These rituals mattered—our tribes cared about them just like they cared about hunting and gathering. But as societies became first agrarian and then industrial, the ecstatic rituals were slowly suppressed or abandoned.

But even as the rituals were abandoned, our ancestors still celebrated.

They celebrated a lot. In the Middle Ages, there were so many holidays, festivals, and carnivals that so-called peasants worked 150 days or fewer each year. They spent the other 215 or so days celebrating. (You still think you're getting enough vacation days?)

Here's something else to consider. The epidemic known as depression (or "melancholy," as it used to be called) was almost unheard of until society suppressed its celebrations and carnivals. The anxiety epidemic followed closely on the heels of depression. Primitive people can't even understand what depression might mean. The closest they can get when anthropologists try to explain it to them is to say, "But wouldn't you hurt yourself then?"

An obsession with sex and sexual purity also showed up when celebrations got suppressed. My hypothesis is that as we lost touch with celebrations and ecstatic dance, sex took on outsized importance. Sex shouldn't be that big a deal. It's only considered a big deal because that's the only activity in modern society in which many people allow themselves to let loose, to reach an emotional climax.

Today we do have rock concerts, sporting competitions, and giant political rallies—probably the closest experiences we have to the celebrations our ancestors participated in. However, most people can't regularly attend concerts or games due to the expense. Also, these modern events are so focused on a tiny group of exalted celebrities.

As you imagine ways to energize your families, groups, and organizations, consider why sporting events, concerts, and rallies are so powerful. Look at how emotional energy builds through rituals.

Take a football game. It's a ritual from start to finish. Announcements boom through the speakers as the crowd arrives. Cheers greet the players as they exit the locker room and run onto the field. The national anthem is sung. The coin toss builds anticipation for the kickoff. Then the game itself begins. Even if you are watching on television, you are to some extent participating in all these rituals. On top of that, you and your friends who are watching together probably have game day rituals like sharing a mound of hot wings and high fiving when your team scores a touchdown.

Sports, concerts, and rallies are wonderful. However, I'd like to see people participate in more rituals like dancing, singing, and storytelling, which don't require a central celebrity.

Tell Your Story

Even the healthiest families sometimes veer off course. Healthy families reinvigorate positive momentum by returning to their core vision, values, and sense of purpose. The family's vision is best communicated as a story.

Maybe the strongest example I've ever seen of using a story to create a compelling mission statement comes from Tom Bilyeu, my best friend going way back to my school days. Tom co-founded Quest Nutrition after financial success in another business left him feeling unsatisfied. When he started the new business, he knew there had to be more to this venture than the desire for profit. He needed to create a business he cared about.

Some of Tom's family members were morbidly obese. His mother, whom he loved deeply, particularly suffered from an unhealthy diet. Tom knew preaching to people about their health wouldn't work. He knew people were used to fast food and processed snacks. He had to find a way to make healthy snacks as delicious as candy bars and potato chips. He didn't know how to do it. He didn't care. He had to figure it out.

As he built Quest, he kept telling that story about his family, his mother, and his mission. He often said the mission of Quest was to end metabolic disease. That's a big mission, which is good because big missions inspire people. Tom's story motivated him, and it motivated everyone around him. His story helped energize and unify the people who worked for Quest. And especially in the early days, it even gave Quest's customers good reasons to want to buy the products.

Eventually Quest became an enormous company, a unicorn among startups. I don't think it could have grown that big so quickly without its powerful sense of purpose.

Never be afraid to tell your story, or to take on a big mission. That might be what you are called to do. No matter how big or small your mission, you make progress with every specific, intentional step toward your goal. It's those small steps that matter anyway, so there is no reason to skimp on the mission or downplay your story.

When you believe your story, and tell it with passion and conviction, your entire group can coalesce around it. The story itself creates emotional energy. Groups of people, families of all kinds, and all types of organizations need a unifying story in order to create the emotional energy that allows everyone to thrive.

And when we hear family stories, we can often see ourselves in the roles. Also, being a storyteller is a role, and so is being a listener. My mother always said part of the purpose of family reunions is to rehearse the family stories. In any healthy family, telling the story is a ritual.

This is why we never fully let go of simple rituals like getting around a campfire and telling tales. In most cultures, the power of stories is well understood. But too many of us modern folks have lost the art. We instead communicate in passive-aggressive corporate-speak, or we try to dominate conversations. We need to get back to telling and listening to stories.

If you feel rusty as a storyteller, don't feel bad. Your culture hasn't taught you well. Go ahead and practice telling your story in your own psychological backstage. That's how I learned to be successful before I became successful. It's how I learned to listen to other people when I didn't yet know how.

I practiced in my head, privately in my room. Some stories, like the one that starts this chapter (about the man with no emotions), healed me even when I just practiced them in my head. They healed me before I told them to anyone else.

The Power of Storytelling

I tell so many stories because I learned a long time ago, in prison ministry, that trying to prove points doesn't always get through to people. But stories do. This is probably why Jesus used parables to teach. It's easier for us to see ourselves in stories because we can imagine playing certain roles. On the other hand, when someone tries to persuade or convince, it often feels as though they are trying to dominate. The natural reaction is defensiveness.

When I share a story, especially one that describes my own shortcomings, failures, or embarrassments, it lowers that defensiveness. It gives listeners permission to admit their own truths. When I can talk about how I overcame my obstacles, listeners gain insight as they imagine themselves overcoming their own obstacles.

Stories are excellent learning tools in any domain, not just when it comes to moral education or personal empowerment. In my experience, one story is better than a thousand conjectures, better than a million ideas.

When I confront a potentially life-changing decision, I do not try to figure it out alone. I find people who have encountered something similar, and I say, "Tell me your story." After I hear a few real, concrete stories, the answer becomes obvious.

For instance, when I started my own business, I talked to a local economist who had been in business for decades. He told me when he started out, he had a contract in hand that made him more money than he had ever made in his life. But after the contract ended, he had great difficulty finding new clients. He was in so much trouble that his bank account was down to $24.72 before the next offer came in. "I still have that banking slip," he told me. He also said, "Make sure you get a nice office. You're going to be spending a lot of time there."

He was right about the office and the risk. My first year in business, I lost money. I almost ran out of savings. I had nightmares for the first time since childhood. And I am also incredibly thankful that I was smart enough to spend twice as much on my office as I spent on my apartment rent during those first few years. I mean, I wasn't spending time in my apartment anyway other than to sleep, and nightmares don't feel any better in a more expensive room.

The economist's story definitely helped me. It may also have helped him. It reminded him of how he rose to become an independent businessperson. It may also have helped him heal from the stress he experienced back then.

Stories are healers. Whenever you tell your story, someone will be healed by hearing it. And it doesn't matter what your story is—anorexia, depression, hallucinations, alcoholism, addiction, abusive relationships, prison time, financial failure, divorce, suicidal thoughts, or whatever. It also doesn't matter whether you tell it as a cry for help, an uplifting tale of recovery, or a simple statement that you feel terrible today.

As long as you tell your story without blaming anyone (including yourself), your story shows someone, somewhere, that they are not alone. Your story shows someone that they can stop feeling ashamed, stop keeping secrets, and start speaking their own truth.

There's no way to know who will be healed by your story. It may be the person who is most like you because they see themselves reflected in shared experiences. Or the person who gets healed might be the least like you because your story doesn't provoke defensiveness.

Our stories are our power and our freedom. Our stories allow us to unite with others and create a sense of purpose in our families.

A Word about Love and Going After What You Really Want

Unfortunately, many people don't recognize the emotional energy created by rituals and unifying stories. Too many folks are burdened with concepts of selfishness. Too many are afraid of ambition, drive, and purpose. Here's the truth. You cannot love others unless you go after what you really want, and you can't go after what you really want without loving others.

Remember that emotions are more contagious than any virus. If I am resentful, then I will spread that resentment without even realizing it. But if a friend is energetic, I get energized simply by being around them. People who pursue their most profound desires often exude energy, excitement, and purpose. People who neglect their own values are at best depressed and anxious, and at worst display a low-grade resentment.

This has certainly been true in my own life. For quite some time, I tried to tell myself my depression affected only me. But my depression affected everyone close to me, everyone in my various emotional families. That all changed when I started pursuing my deepest purpose.

When I go after what I really want, the people closest to me change. When I pursue my deepest goals, other family members are more likely to feel they have unspoken permission to do the same. When I say no to things that do not fit my values, other people feel they have permission to say no.

The secret, the incredibly difficult balancing act, is to clearly define yourself and your goals while staying connected to others. This is a necessary balancing act because unless your goals are limited, you won't be able to get there alone. You will need to love others—or at least be incredibly good at faking it.

Loving others is not just a feeling. Loving someone means respecting them—especially when they disappoint, anger, or frustrate you. It means listening to them when they tell you what it means to love them instead of doing for them what you wish someone else would do for you. Loving others means listening so closely that you could speak from their position if you had to.

Going after what you really want means first admitting what you want—and admitting you might not be skilled enough yet to achieve it. It means knowing you are going to fail and fail often. It means taking tiny steps toward your goals and celebrating each and every small victory along the way.

Now I want to talk about what happens when you don't go after what you really want. When I look back at times when I was controlling, those situations had one thing in common: I wasn't pursuing my own life. I was going after what someone else wanted, even if they had never made their desires explicit. But I knew, consciously or not. Since I was pursuing someone else's dreams, my efforts were forced, painful, and labored. That energy rubbed off on other people. They didn't want to get involved, so I tried to manipulate them. This led to anxiety, burnout, and stress, which of course led to more controlling behavior on my part.

These three things go hand in hand: (1) setting boundaries, (2) pursuing your own life, and (3) not controlling others. If you don't say no to people, you won't have the energy to live your own life. If you don't have that energy, people aren't drawn to you, because there's nothing positive to attract them. So you use your remaining emotional energy trying to control others, which backfires. You end up feeling stretched out, thin, and brittle.

You might even end up with a victim complex, feeling like you are always doing things for everyone else. And a victim complex leads to envy, entitlement, and abusive behavior.

Speaking of envy, here is a widely reported truth about the human condition. Most people are happier making $80,000 per year if everyone else around them is making $70,000, than they are making $90,000 per year if everyone else is making $100,000. Numerous studies have shown that controlling for all other factors, people are unhappy if they live in a neighborhood where their neighbors make more money than they do.

But here is a less widely reported truth. People who make $70,000 in a year are vastly less likely to care what anyone else is making if they made $65,000 last year. They feel so good about moving forward that they don't need to covet their neighbor's salary. That feeling of forward progress stops envy in its tracks.

Forward momentum also can provide emotional health to any family, even one that is in statistical decline, such as a church or organization that is older and shrinking. The group can still create momentum by repeating a few powerful habits. First, remember the family's story, the mission. Define clear, reachable goals that fit the mission. Then move toward achieving those goals. Every time positive action is taken, celebrate. Even in a declining family, consistent steps forward will create momentum and emotional energy.

Real emotional energy pushes envy, listlessness, and self-sabotage out of the group. A unifying mission creates goals for the whole family to pursue. A powerful story energizes everyone. And forward progress on small goals is always good, even if you never reach your stated long-term goal. In fact, on a day-to-day level, the emotional energy gleaned from making progress with others is itself the goal.

Purpose, ambition, and leadership are beautiful because it's wonderful to be in a family that has a uniting story. It's awesome when the whole family works together to advance the family's mission, and there is always a deep well of emotional energy to draw from. Even better than being in one healthy family, though, is being part of many healthy families.

The Path to Rationality Is through Diverse Families

I once lived with a hippy in a house full of college students. The hippy was all into peace, love, and togetherness.

He was also a Seattle Mariners fan. I sat down with him once while he was watching a game. Omar Vizquel, a shortstop for the opposing Cleveland Indians, made a seemingly impossible catch. I yelled, "That was amazing!"

This peace-loving hippy jumped up from his chair, enraged. He was shaking. He pointed his finger at me and said, "I just can't handle this. I'm gonna have to ask you to leave. I can't watch this game with you cheering for the other team."

I thought, *Wow. So much for peace, love, and unity. Just don't mess with his Mariners, I guess.*

I've often noticed that people are magically blind to when their team cheats. But when the other team cheats, it's some sort of ethical apocalypse. People often have completely different standards for those on the opposing side.

This is all part of a larger truth: most of us feel the emotion first, then we construct some rationalization to justify the emotion. A lot of times, the rationalizations involve supporting the team or defending our friends. Or even worse, we're defending our social circle in our heads. In the worst-case scenario, we are defending our past selves in long-ago arguments.

Believe it or not, I am going to suggest that the solution to this problem is *not* to become more rational. It won't work. My brain always wants to act in the best interest of the family or the tribe, whether I like it or not. And my brain does not like to admit my tribe is wrong.

The solution is to make more friends who are totally removed from my current circles of friends—totally different teams, different tribes, and different families. Then I can cheer for brilliant athleticism instead of just rooting for one side.

I used to believe that science advances because individual scientists are rational. Oh, no, scientists are just as irrational as everyone else. They get attached to their theories and don't want to admit their theories are false. Meanwhile, other scientists have competing theories to which they are equally irrationally attached. And what do these irrational scientists do while clinging to their theories? They dig up every fact they can to support their ideas. They come up with every plausible analysis to support their conclusions. And then they go to war.

When the next generation of scientists comes up, they see all these facts that have been discovered. Then it's clear to them which theories are better. The next generation rationally decides between the theories or else synthesizes the competing theories into a superior idea.

Life as a whole is a lot like that.

I wish I could say you can just think your way to being wiser, more intelligent, or more rational. But it won't happen. You have to let competing ideas—about happiness, money, culture, exercise, diet, friendship, relationships, business, values, romance, children, religion, and more—go to war in your head. You won't let it happen unless you're willing to root for competing ideas. And you'll root for those ideas only if you have true friends who genuinely believe them.

For instance, I didn't understand my own values about money until I had groups of friends that were rich, poor, middle-class, working-class, students worried about debt, and business owners worried about costs. Only then did I stop clinging to beliefs about money that were handed down to me from my parents.

If you are suffering needlessly, you have beliefs or ideas that are false, harmful, or self-defeating. My self-defeating ideas did not go away by thinking my way through them. They went away only when I associated with people who disagreed with them and became such close friends with those people that I started to root for their ideas and beliefs.

And I don't worry that you will associate with the wrong crowd or get the wrong ideas. I know you will do that. I did that. Along the way to getting better, you will sometimes get temporarily worse. But taking risks is a necessary step if you want to uncover all the facts relevant to your own life. You have to emotionally connect with contradictory ideas in order for outdated beliefs to fall apart and your old self to collapse. After the collapse, you can judge your beliefs and values based on evidence, rather than clinging to them just because they were handed down to you.

I have an absurd story to share about online video game drama. I used to be quite into World of Warcraft. In WoW (as it's abbreviated), I had to join a guild in order to engage with the game's best content. So here I am in this guild called Clan Meteorites or something, in an online game, with a bunch of people I have never met in real life and never will. In this game, my character was a healing wizard-type named Backleshark.

One day, a married couple who always played together got into a huge argument with the guild leader. After hours of agonizing over how to handle the situation, I got involved. I sided with the married couple because I felt they were being treated unfairly. The argument raged over the internet, and I quit the guild, but only after getting so stressed out that I nearly became depressed. The conflict dominated my waking thoughts for about a week. I probably dreamed about it.

After I left the guild, I continued to play online games with some of my friends from Clan Meteorites. But as the years passed, they drifted out of my life. I am no longer connected with any of them. At one time, I cared so much about their opinions and arguments. Now they don't even exist.

As the online video game guild dissolved, so did the old conflicts. I find it strange that when I was inside the conflict, I couldn't see that someday none of it would matter. My lack of perspective seems bizarre to me now, especially given that this wasn't even the real world. It wasn't my world at all. It was Backleshark's world, a world of goblins and sorcery, and it could never have lasted. Why couldn't I see that the group of people whose opinions I cared about so much would someday just be part of a weird story I barely remember?

Here are two things I wish someone had told me decades ago. First, my circle of friends now won't be my circle of friends forever. Someday, I may not care about these people at all, and I should act accordingly. Second, I need more than one circle of friends. Any group of friends can become toxic, and if I only have one group, how do I know if it's the group that's toxic or if I am?

I had always thought I was a rational, logical, and self-interested individual. But the experience of joining diverse families showed me I had been clinging to outdated ideas. Once I intentionally kept multiple circles of friends who did not know one another and who did not share the same beliefs or values, I was surprised to see my own true values emerge.

CHAPTER 8

HOW TO TRANSFORM YOUR EMOTIONAL REALITY

In a healthy family, you can accelerate the long process of intergenerational health by changing your emotional habits. You can redefine what it means to "win" and turn even your most negative emotions into powerful allies.

I HAVE A CLOSE FRIEND WHO IS A RECOVERING ADDICT. Every chance she gets, she posts on social media that she has one more day, clean and sober. Every time there is something mathematically interesting about how many days, months, or years she's been sober, she posts about it. She publicly celebrates it. And she expects her friends to celebrate too.

Learn from her.

My friend is changing her emotional definition of what it means to win. In the past, winning for her was about dominating arguments, feeling more beautiful than other women, or settling grudges. Now, winning is about having one more sober day.

That's a powerful, beautiful definition of victory. The key is that it's an emotional definition. She feels it. It's not just an idea she tries to believe in.

Accept the Truth about Your Pettiest Emotions

It's time to talk about some uncomfortable facts about myself. I suffer from pretty serious mental illnesses. For instance, the other day I was attacked by bats in my house. There were no bats. This is a normal experience for me—I have hallucinated and heard voices my whole life. I function just fine as long as I stay centered and don't overreact.

To survive, I've had to confront, analyze, and understand my darkest, strangest, and least admirable emotions. It has been difficult, often soul crushing. That's how I noticed that winning and losing seem to matter a great deal to me, even with the most trivial things.

When I was a child, my father noticed I got excessively aggravated if I failed to do well at an arcade game. I figured it was just because I was young. But even now, while playing games on my phone, if I do poorly, I sometimes cry. It doesn't happen often, but it does happen.

At some point, I decided to be ruthlessly honest with myself about my reactions to issues that are important. And I noticed some awful truths about myself. Even when I do wrong or make a terrible mistake, as long as I perceive myself as the winner in the interaction, I'm not bothered about my missteps or wrongdoings. Even when I treat people badly, I don't feel bad about it as long as it seems I won the conflict. Furthermore, I don't remain angry with people unless I lose the conflict, even when they are outright abusive toward me.

I tried to figure out how to change this aspect of myself. I asked myself, *How do I stop caring so much about winning and losing?* I got nowhere with that. It turned into a self-centered, navel-gazing exercise. Eventually though, I came up with a better question: *How can I change my emotional definition of winning?*

I started asking this question after I learned that, when getting out of debt, it's often best to pay off your smallest debts first. Then you have a small victory to celebrate. In celebrating that victory, you make further victories more likely.

I remember the first time I worked with a client on paying down debt. This client had two credit cards with outstanding balances. One was large and had a higher interest rate. The other was much smaller and could be paid off within a year. Now mathematically, it made more sense to pay off the larger debt first. But I knew better. I recommended she first pay off the small debt. "You need a victory," I told her.

The next time I saw her she told me that, for the most part, her summer had been a total disaster. She had to work massive overtime and barely got to enjoy the sunshine. But there was one bright spot—that credit card she paid down. "Remember when you told me I needed a victory? Paying off that card was the one bright spot to my whole summer! When I paid off the card, I didn't cut it up. Instead I sealed it in an envelope and covered the envelope with glitter and crayon markings that read, '*Now, do you really want to open this envelope again?*'"

I thought, *Glitter. Glitter, really? Yes, this woman has it right!*

Then I had one of the strangest spiritual experiences of my life. I felt God was telling me to go to the casino. I could not figure out why. I don't gamble. I don't drink or smoke. The all-you-can-eat buffets were fun, but why was God calling me to the casino? Was I supposed to preach there?

Then one day in Vegas, I saw someone win at craps. Lord, were they screamin' and hollerin'. That's when it hit me. *What if I were to celebrate my small victories like that? What if I were to celebrate every blessing in my life? What if I were to celebrate my friends' victories with that much intensity?*

Then I realized I didn't even have to wait for results. I could celebrate taking action and doing right.

Anytime I connect with or uplift someone who is sick, isolated, incarcerated, or unhappy, I celebrate. Anytime I act ethically in the face of temptation or peer pressure, I celebrate. Anytime I do something healthy, like exercise, I celebrate. Anytime I defeat procrastination by taking action, I celebrate.

And when I say "celebrate," I mean that, at least in my mind, I celebrate like people do in Las Vegas when they hit a jackpot. I celebrate like people do when their team wins the Super Bowl. Hey, in public, I don't go too crazy, but I go crazy in my head. And in private, I go all out!

The constant celebrations have changed how I emotionally define winning. And that changes the story I tell about myself and thus, my identity. So now when I do what's right or defeat procrastination, I actually feel like a winner. And these personal battles occur far more often than interpersonal conflicts. I still encounter conflicts. But as with my hallucinations, those conflicts don't take hold of me the way they used to, and their grip fades quickly.

Procrastination

Speaking of procrastination, let's discuss writing this book. At first, I procrastinated. Then, I followed some advice from Ray Bradbury. I just started writing. I didn't care whether or not it was any good or if I wrote very much. But every single day, I wrote. It didn't matter if I wrote only one word, one sentence, one paragraph, or one page. I just wrote. As soon as I wrote anything, I celebrated. I patted myself on the back.

Well, once I start writing, I might as well keep writing. Our brains don't like to let things go once we start. That's why constant interruptions like social media can be so damaging. Once we start looking at Facebook, we don't want to stop.

Just like a recovering addict—a recovering Facebook addict maybe?—I took things one step at a time. *Just write something.* Celebrating that simple step changed my emotional definition of winning. After I got used to writing every day, I increased my expectations slightly. I made a note on my phone's calendar as to whatever I thought needed the most attention in the book. If I did any work at all on what I'd noted—*anything*, no matter how simple—I celebrated. I then deleted the notification, which cleared my mind.

As time went on, I found that I had a hard time shutting down the Word document once I opened it. Writing my book had actually become addictive. As I celebrated each small victory, and as the months passed, it got to the point where I thought about the book all the time, just like I thought obsessively about video games when I was young.

I used to be unable to put my phone down and stop texting during an argument. Now it's easy. I used to obsess over vengeful thoughts. Now I forget them. I used to hate seeing my rivals succeed. Now I focus on my own success.

I am still petty. I care enormously about winning and losing. But now I emotionally define victory in a healthy way.

In the past, I had emotionally defined winning as either big successes in the far-off future or as dominance of other people. But people usually resent being dominated. Dominance may have gotten me a temporary control-freak high, but it never moved me an inch closer to health, love, success, financial independence, or happiness.

Meanwhile, focusing on things I have no control over eventually leads to misery. Even if, for a while, I make extraordinary progress toward my big, far-off goals, someday my luck might run out. And if that happens when my focus has been on things I cannot control, I will crash and burn. This is to say nothing of the fact that big successes are so far away in the future that I won't get a quick enough emotional payoff anyway.

So the good news is that you can use your pettiest impulses to achieve extraordinary goals. If you can successfully define winning as taking small steps forward, you will feel compelled to do what's necessary—much the same way a Facebook addiction compels someone to check their notifications every ten minutes. You will find that you can't help but do the right thing, just like I am as I stand here at my computer and write. I was going to quit, but I can't let it go. It is like an addiction, and that is wonderful. Yes, you can get addicted to doing the right thing.

Your emotions don't always have your best interests at heart, in large part because many emotional responses are still living in the world as it existed ten thousand years ago. But no matter how outdated, petty, or trivial your emotions are, they can be harnessed to push you in the right direction.

Little day-to-day celebrations give you an immediate emotional payoff. The big stuff, the grand commitments, the high-flown speeches—they aren't likely to change who you are right now. They may inspire you, but inspiration is often fleeting.

Create Emotional Energy by Celebrating Small Victories

Remember these key factors:

1. We all make decisions with our emotions.
2. Those emotions are often incredibly petty.
3. The pettiness can usually be defined as "winning" or "losing," in the crudest sense.
4. When you celebrate small victories, you change what winning and losing means to you.
5. Changing your emotional definition of winning and losing changes your unconscious choices, and gets you addicted to staying the course on a positive path.
6. That positive addiction transforms your unconscious identity, leading to changed relationships with everyone around you.

Once your relationships start changing, your families can start getting healthier and it all becomes a virtuous cycle. That family health will get passed down through the generations to people you might never meet.

Throughout this chapter I talk about changing your emotional definition of victory from an individual perspective. But the transformation is even more powerful when the whole family participates. Consider this summary:

1. We all make decisions with our emotions.
2. Emotions—positive and negative—are more contagious than any virus.
3. Celebrating small victories produces emotional energy, which is so contagious that on a group level it turns into momentum. That momentum revitalizes the entire group.
4. When you focus on the healthiest members of a family

or group, their emotional energy attracts other healthy people and also gives everyone in the family something to aspire to, enjoy, and participate in.

5. The least healthy members, who are no longer the focus, now have examples to look up to. But they also have enough emotional energy to take on the risks, pain, and uncertainty of growth. The group has momentum, so now they feed off of it.

Consider a church that wants to grow. There might be discussion about the best way to present the church to its community. That conversation is fine, but what attracts people to any family is the emotional energy of its members. And what builds that energy is when the group returns to its mission, sets achievable short-term goals, and then celebrates actions taken to move toward those goals. The church will bring on more members by celebrating its purposeful actions than by focusing on how to attract new people—especially if the lack of new members is considered a problem.

This same principle works for all types of families, organizations, and relationships. It's always better to focus on the core values, beliefs, or mission. Set achievable goals and celebrate taking actions that move the group toward those goals. Focusing on even the smallest goals is better than focusing on perceived problems or long-term results.

Many groups, though, are so used to celebrating only results, and that is a dead end. To build momentum, the emotional definition of victory has to be transformed. It's so important to change how you emotionally define a win, because I doubt it's possible to not care about winning and losing.

The Terror of Losing

Once, when I was in a deep depression, I went to a club to listen to music. I couldn't get excited about it. I ended up sitting on a couch. A woman sat next to me. The music was loud. I guess she was talking to me. I didn't have the energy to respond. Suddenly, I realized she was hitting on me. I said some version of "no."

She stood up and screamed, "You just think you're so much better than everyone else! You won't even let me buy you a drink? Seriously? Like how hard is it to accept a drink from a woman? My God!" Finally, after about ten minutes of her ranting, one of her embarrassed friends escorted her out.

When I was much younger, I moved in with a woman I thought was looking for a roommate. She was looking for more than that, though, and she threatened me with a gun after I refused to have sex with her. It was the only time anyone's ever threatened my life over the issue, but it is one of several times my overly literal, autistic self just didn't understand sex was an assumed part of the deal.

Now I'll share a story about someone else—a pastor who always seemed angry when he preached. It was unclear to me and everyone else as to why he was so mad. His sermons were uncomfortable. One day I was talking with a member of the congregation about the angry pastor. I mentioned that the pastor was opposed to gay marriage, but his affiliated religious organization had chosen to accept it. The other member responded, "So, he lost."

Yes, I realized. *He lost.*

Later on, he became even angrier over a different issue. The church had, more than twenty years before, bought a piece of land intended for senior housing. But even at that time, they had been told the land could not be zoned for that purpose.

Finally the church decided to sell the land. The pastor was enraged despite the fact that the church had done nothing with the land for two decades and had no realistic future plans either.

The pastor was upset despite the fact that the church needed the money. He was upset despite the fact that no one wanted to take care of the land, and it was mostly an eyesore where people dumped garbage. He was upset despite the fact that selling the land meant it could be used for low-income housing, which the surrounding community desperately needed. But selling the land was admitting defeat. Twenty years seems like a long time to cling to something just to avoid admitting that a loss.

I've watched businesspeople, who know how to be successful, run an idea into the ground by making the same mistakes over and over again. As far as I can tell, they had a painful argument about their big concept and can't stand to admit they were wrong. So now they put more and more effort into something that's never going to work, throwing good money after bad. Clinging to old arguments can be an expensive habit.

I've seen folks stay in dysfunctional relationships, partly because they don't want to admit they made a bad choice. I watch other folks spread rage and anxiety through gossip because they are upset that they lost some status competition. I watch people madly pursue things they don't care about or that would be outright detrimental, mostly because they started pursuing—and now they can't stand to lose the race.

Sometimes, it's as if I were watching people curse at reality itself. Like that woman at the club, except there's no one sitting on the couch to yell at—just some embarrassed friends, wondering if they should intervene.

When I think about how deeply important winning is to some people, even in trivial competitions, it's hard for me to imagine how such an ingrained feature of human interrelationship can be eliminated. But energy can always be redirected.

Stop "Should"ing All Over Yourself

A lot of us are plagued by notions of what we "should" do. But we don't necessarily know or remember where these notions came from. All we know is that we *should* do whatever it is, and if we don't do it, we must be unproductive or selfish. An acquaintance of mine calls this "'should'ing all over myself."

A year or so after the pandemic began, a friend told me COVID-19 might have saved his life. Now before you get angry, he wasn't referring to the disease. He was talking about how, due to the social changes during the pandemic, he had stopped doing all sorts of things he thought he had to do. And he learned that most of those things didn't matter. It was liberating. In fact, it probably saved him from a crushing depression.

I have been thinking a lot about his story.

I've also been thinking about a *Star Wars* game I used to play on my phone. (There's a connection here, believe it or not.) I eventually decided to quit this game because of my unhealthy attachment to it. The game requires players to log on at certain times of the day in order to maximize its activities. I noticed I was often thinking about when to log on. I would realize the time and think, *Oh, I have to log on now*.

Wait. I...*have to* log on? Where did that come from? It's a game. Why do I *have to* do something?

Then I noticed that logging on at specified times was chopping up my day into little pieces. See, if you want to do what I call "deep work" (like writing a book), you can't let your day get chopped up into pieces. It interrupts focus. You can't let yourself get distracted by emails, texts, phone calls, or social media. You can't constantly interrupt yourself with mundane tasks or interpersonal drama.

This phone game was distracting. It was interrupting my day, chopping it up, and lowering my productivity. So, I quit. I still play my computer game online because its activities are the same no matter when I log on, so there's no schedule.

I am slowly realizing how important it is that when I started my own business, I refused to set an alarm clock, refused to allow myself to do busywork, and refused to let myself get interrupted by texts and emails. Many people tell themselves they are working hard when they are just distracting themselves with busywork.

During the COVID-19 lockdown, I eliminated everything from my life that didn't seem important. I ditched all contracts and projects that weren't going to produce real value for other people. At first, I thought that not being able to travel would bother me. But after eliminating distractions from my life, I no longer felt the need to go on vacations.

I also no longer need to use video games to escape. In fact, I no longer even enjoy playing video games if I haven't already gotten my writing done for the day. I used to use video games as a reward for doing the right thing. Now, they are just pure entertainment.

Then my food cravings disappeared. I used to reward myself with food when I didn't play video games, and then I'd reward myself by playing video games when I refrained from eating junk food. Both cravings have vanished since I stopped chopping up my day by doing things that don't matter.

I don't believe I was ever successful at lying to myself, at any time in my life. My brain always knew when my work, schedule, priorities, jobs, and projects weren't useful. Of course, my ego didn't like to lose arguments. So it would double down on my useless endeavors by telling me to work harder, show more passion, or convince someone else to join me in my foolishness.

But my brain knew all along. And the real result of spending so much time doing things that didn't matter was that my brain demanded to be soothed, distracted, and numbed with junk food, video games, and vacations.

I noticed a long time ago that my best ideas seemed to come when I was on vacation. I wondered why that was. Now I can see that it's because I wasn't chopping up my day. While vacationing I slept when I was tired, ate when I was hungry, and moved my body when I felt like moving it. Lo and behold, my brain and body were more productive when I wasn't working hard, because working hard is something I don't need to convince myself to do unless my ego is demanding it. And my ego demands hard work only when the work is bunk.

If you suffer from fatigue, brain fog, the need to escape, foolish cravings, burnout, or vague and unsettling stress, consider the possibility that you are "should"-ing all over yourself. Consider the possibility that the many things you think you *should* be doing are chopping up your day and destroying your productivity.

You know those dreams in which you have a homework assignment due, and you forgot to do it? Fifteen years after graduating from college, I had one of those dreams. Fifteen years—and the only thing shocking to me now is that it took so long to realize how much harm chopping up my day with busywork has caused.

But busywork isn't always just busywork. Sometimes busy-work is procrastination, or outright fear.

Procrastination and Narcissism, Fear and Control

Procrastination happens because when you fantasize rather than take action, there is no failure. You are in complete control of your own mental universe, and you are in complete control of the results of every action. So the greater your desire to control results, the more likely you are to procrastinate. For many people, that means the more important something is to them, the more they care about it, the more likely they are to procrastinate.

Procrastination is different from avoidance. We avoid things that are unpleasant. I don't think people procrastinate on doing their taxes—they avoid doing their taxes. Artists and entrepreneurs, on the other hand, procrastinate on precisely the projects they are most passionate about.

I defeated procrastination by celebrating small victories. Eventually, my mind came to emotionally identify success as action. Taking action was a victory, while failure was just inaction. And I dislike failure. Once I started celebrating taking action instead of celebrating results, my desire to control others subsided. In fact, my need to control anything at all subsided, and procrastination disappeared.

There are lots of things that cannot be controlled, like the results of a specific action or the consequences of any given risk. Something else that cannot be controlled is what other people think of you. Attempting to control others' thoughts or beliefs leads to narcissism—a condition even nastier than procrastination.

I call narcissism the most insidious addiction: being

addicted to feeling special or important instead of feeling loved. It is so insidious that in many families it is encouraged, and everyone thinks they are doing the right thing by encouraging it. Almost everyone I know who suffers from this addiction doesn't even realize they are addicted.

For the purposes of this section on narcissism, I define "addiction" as craving something even though it no longer provides pleasure or satisfaction. Everyone wants to feel special, unique, important, or powerful sometimes. That's not the issue. The issue is when you still crave that feeling even after it has stopped giving you any satisfaction. When you crave feeling special or important like I used to crave ice cream even after I couldn't taste it anymore because my mouth had gone numb from the cold.

This addiction to feeling special or important instead of feeling loved undermined me for most of my adult life. It isolated me and was one of the underlying causes of my fifteen-year-long clinical depression. I believe that the addiction to feeling important is an epidemic that sabotages many people I most care about.

I lived most of my life with no awareness of my own addiction to feeling great, special, or important. (Probably because I wasn't great or important. But see, there's no connection between feeling important and being important.)

Depression Is Not an Excuse

I've noticed a troubling, disturbing trend. People are using their mental illnesses as excuses for their narcissistic or even abusive behavior. Folks, that's not acceptable. I'll use clinical depression as an example because that is what I lived through. I'll also return to the subject of abusive behavior because that's the worst-case scenario for what the addiction to feeling special or important might lead to.

Abusive behavior causes depression—not the other way around. Let me explain. Anger comes with a burst of adrenaline that temporarily increases confidence and vitality. It's emotional energy, but it's only a short-term chemical high. Afterward, there is a slump.

So whenever you use anger to energize yourself, you borrow from your future store of emotional energy. And you cannot keep borrowing forever. Eventually, the debt must be paid. The debt is paid with that numb, lifeless feeling that becomes so familiar. But you can still get that hit of anger by replaying events, over and over again, in your head. Every time you remember the bad things people have done to you—the insults, the humiliations—you get angry. Anger makes you feel alive, temporarily. Then the slump comes again. You need a stronger dose of adrenaline.

You get an even stronger dose of adrenaline by talking with friends about the terrible things people have done to you. Your friends egg you on. They encourage you. It feels good. You're the victim in your own story. You're the Hollywood underdog fighting back against the bad guys. That adrenaline surge of anger feels good.

But then you're alone, and the familiar numbness of depression returns. You need more anger.

You've learned that people blindly support you when you're the victim. It feels good to think life is a movie and you're the main character. You go online and read about narcissism and borderline personality, or whatever disorder you stumble across. Now, it's not enough to talk about what people did. Now, you need to diagnose and label them. They are no longer just people who did bad things. Now, they are bad people.

So you ascribe devious intentions to compassionate actions. As long as you talk about intentions, which are invisible, you can tell whatever fabricated story you want about anyone. Now, you replay conversations in your head, taking phrases way out of context. You are angry every time you remember what someone said, because you needed the adrenaline from that hit of anger. And your anger poisons every memory.

Your poisoned memories allow you to blow other people's behavior out of proportion while you ignore your own. You ignore your cold shoulders, your stonewalling, your loud sighs, your condescending tone, your intimidating anger, your character-assassinating gossip, your attempts to isolate the person, your threats to harm yourself, your constant provocations, your alcohol abuse, your crossing of physical boundaries, your bullying, your criticism, and your contempt.

You ignore your blame. Instead, needing more and more of that anger-induced adrenaline, you focus on the most minor slights, real or imagined. It is always someone or something else's fault. And eventually, you define affronts to your ego as "harm."

You read some self-help and learn that you deserve love. But your idea of love is that other people give you what you want. Or your culture tells you that you deserve respect. But respect to you means that other people submit. You believe you are entitled to the blind support your friends gave you when you first told them, angrily, about the bad things people have done to you. You believe you are entitled due to your victim status—no wait, you are told not to use the word "victim." You're entitled due to your "survivor" status.

But every time you replay the insults in your head, every time you gossip so your friends hear only your version of the movie, every time you lash out with threats or even physical

violence, every time you use anger to get that burst of power...
the darkness returns.

Anger doesn't make you powerful. It only makes you feel
powerful, temporarily. When the anger fades, the numbness
of depression returns, even worse than last time. You are not
abusive because you're depressed. You are depressed because
you're abusive.

If this applies to you or to someone you love, there is a way
out. Remember why anger exists. It has a positive function.

I get angry so I can defend the tribe against sabretooth
tigers. I get angry so that I can transform into the Mandalorian
and defend Baby Yoda. I get angry so I can protect those I love.

But here in the twenty-first century, no one needs protection from sabretooth tigers. The Baby Yodas that surround me
don't need me to battle death troopers. They need protection
from a sick culture that tells them they are special and important—and deserve to be treated as such—but does not teach
them how to love or be loved.

Anger makes me feel powerful. But connecting with other
human beings makes me powerful, regardless of how I feel, as
does pursuing my own goals and living up to my core values.

So every time I feel the need to use anger for an adrenaline burst, I take it as a signal. Instead of wallowing in anger,
I connect with someone. I see them in person, text-message
them, or respond to them on social media. It doesn't matter
whether or not they reply. I get to work on something I care
about. And particularly in a social setting, I remind myself that
the more I am tempted to use anger, the more important it is
to set a positive example instead.

It does not matter how important or big an action is.
Habits don't change through grand gestures. They change
through the consistent implementation of small actions. I

have interrupted my anger addiction hundreds of times, and yes, I celebrated every time. That's what it takes. Addictions are hard to undo. Old habits must be replaced by new ones.

If you are addicted to anger, as I was once, here's my promise to you.

Interrupt that anger five hundred times by connecting, protecting, working hard, or setting an example. Interrupt that surge of anger the moment you remember that you have a choice. Do it often enough and your depression will disappear.

You will *be* powerful instead of feeling powerful.

There is nothing special about anger, narcissism, or depression. This method of interruption works with most mental illnesses and emotional addictions.

Anyone Can Change

No more excuses, because even psychopaths can change their brain structure. If a psychopath can change, so can you.

Neuroscientist Kent Kiehl has made it his life's mission to study psychopathy. He was one of the first researchers to use mobile brain scanners to analyze the differences in the brains of psychopaths. He started a program at the Mendota Juvenile Treatment Center, which works with criminal offenders who were deemed uncontrollable at other institutions.

Punishment is usually ineffective when dealing with psychopaths, so Dr. Kiehl's team focused on rewards. They gave the young men in the juvenile center small rewards for any form of good behavior, no matter how trivial. The rewards also scaled up over time as behavior improved.

The researchers then followed the three hundred men they worked with and compared results to a similar group of psychopaths who had not participated in the rewards program.

After five years, the results were astonishing—a 50 percent reduction in violent crime compared to the control group and a 34 percent reduction in recidivism. But it wasn't just their behavior that changed. Their brains changed. Dr. Kiehl and his team continue to study the changes in the young men's brains to see what can be learned.

No matter who you are or what your circumstances might be, you can change your behavior, which in turn changes your brain and thus your thought patterns and emotions. Anyone can do it. It makes no difference what you were born with, what label someone tagged you with, what mental illnesses you might have, or what your genetics are. You can change your brain and thus your genetic code. Those changes will be handed down from generation to generation in ways that neither you nor anyone else can predict.

Some people think they are too old to change. I was surprised by current research being done on rats. Researchers have found, to their shock, that the brains of older rats are more malleable than younger ones. That's what makes it harder for changes to take hold, oddly. It requires more repetition to create a new default neural pathway, because an older brain changes too easily.

If you feel like behavioral change is harder as you get older, maybe you are carrying around old arguments and family triangles. Emotional junk has built up. The conversations in your head have built up. Maybe you have started to believe the labels other people have put on you. You've adopted an identity, and that identity governs your behavior. It's not that you're older and biologically incapable of change. It's that you are carrying around too much baggage, and it's too easy to revert to what you're used to.

But you can let go of all of it; you can change anything.

Positive change might mean letting go of who you think you are, which means letting go of your ego. That's OK, because you are not your ego. Your ego acts like you can't live without it, but in reality, it is holding you back.

The Truth about Self-Sabotage

Your ego is a reflection of other people's observations of you, so your ego should stick to observing. It should take control only for short periods of time. But your ego likes to be in charge. When it tries to stay in charge, the day-to-day you, the real you, rebels. And that's self-sabotage.

For instance, my ego might tell me I should date someone more beautiful, own a bigger house, make more money at a more prestigious job, or go on a vendetta against some jerk who was mean to me once back in third grade. But do any of these goals fit with the day-to-day me, who cares so much about cleanliness and financial stability? Or do these goals just come from my ego reflecting other people's expectations?

Because if these goals don't match who I am, the day-to-day me will rebel against my ego. The result is pure misery—misery for me, and misery for those around me.

Let me be more specific about what I mean when I say the "day-to-day me," or "who I am." This does not refer to who I tell myself I am. This is who I am even if I don't realize or admit it. My behavior and immediate unconscious reactions demonstrate the day-to-day me.

According to psychiatrist Steven Reich, research shows there are sixteen different fundamental desires, or values. These are the values of day-to-day me—the desires that I pursue for their own sake, the end goals. All of us prioritize a small number of those sixteen basic desires. And we all have at least one or two desires we don't care about at all. How we combine what we care about and what we don't makes us so different from one another.

Briefly, these are the sixteen basic desires as outlined by Dr. Reich:

1. **Power:** the desire to influence others. Ambition, dominance, leadership.
2. **Independence:** the desire for self-reliance. Resistance to advice, wanting to be on your own.
3. **Curiosity:** the desire for knowledge. Learning for its own sake, asking lots of questions, thinking about what's true.
4. **Acceptance:** the desire for inclusion. Wanting people to like you, to not criticize you.
5. **Order:** the desire for organization. Cleanliness, planning, having rules.
6. **Saving:** the desire to collect things. Hoarding, being tight with money.
7. **Honor:** the desire to be loyal to one's parents and heritage. Being principled and also your relationship with your parents specifically.
8. **Idealism:** the desire for social justice. Volunteering, donating time and money, sacrificing for humanitarian causes.
9. **Social contact:** the desire for companionship. Caring about friends who aren't your parents, kids, or romantic partners. Just liking to have lots of people around.
10. **Family:** the desire to raise one's own children. (Notice that caring about different types of relationships represents different basic desires!)
11. **Status:** the desire for social standing. Wanting expensive things, wanting to impress people, caring about what you're associated with.

12. **Vengeance:** the desire to get even. Competitiveness, revenge, aggression.
13. **Romance:** the desire for sex and beauty. Caring about your sexual relationships or wanting to have lots of them.
14. **Eating:** the desire to consume food. The importance of family dinners and social get-togethers that involve food.
15. **Physical activity:** the desire for the exercise of muscles. Enjoying sports, being outdoorsy.
16. **Tranquility:** the desire for emotional calm. Having high anxiety, being fearful.

The basic desires that matter to you are those you pursue for their own sake, not because they get you something else. I care about four basic desires: honor, independence, order, and curiosity. There are several basic desires I do not care about at all: family, physical activity, tranquility, romance, status, acceptance, and power. The remaining basic desires are things I care about but not as much.

When I pursue any of those basic desires I don't care about, it's only to gain honor, independence, order, or curiosity. So for instance, I dance often. But I don't dance because I love physical activity. I dance because I need to stay healthy in order to be independent. On the other hand, I desire order for its own sake, so when I clean or organize, those activities reflect my basic desires.

Now maybe you care about status, in which case living in a nice house would not be a demand of your ego. It would be a demand of the real, day-to-day you! If you try to live somewhere modest, that's your ego telling you to be humble. (And yes, your ego can tell you to humble yourself.) But for me, since I don't care about status, wanting to live in a nicer house is just some ego trip. Therefore, the same action can be pure egotism for one person and an expression of basic desires for another.

We all have different combinations of basic desires, and those combinations make up our deep values. And we all sabotage ourselves when we follow our ego's wishes instead of our deep values. When I try to ignore the day-to-day me, it rebels. The day-to-day me rebels through procrastination, pointless or fabricated conflict, and a general unwillingness to put forth my best effort.

I once read a commentary from a psychiatrist who compared the ego to an abusive boyfriend. This makes a lot of sense. Your ego tells you that you can't live without him, that all your successes are due to him, but your failures are all your fault...and so on. It is worth thinking about, that our own egos often do act almost as abusive partners.

But just like your pettiest emotions can be channeled into something beautiful and even loving, your ego can become a close friend and steady supporter. When I focus on what's most important, my ego is great at helping me say no to all the distractions. My ego is fantastic at standing up for me when I need it to. And when I ask my ego to do something important, it feels important. Then it calms down a little bit when I need it to.

Since the ego is meant to be an observer, I ask it to help me watch out for signs that I'm regressing into old habits. I also ask my ego to be like a trainer, a coach, to help me stay on course.

Now that I've introduced the day-to-day me and the day-to-day you, let's look at why we all need to be fake sometimes. At first this might seem contradictory. But when learning new emotional definitions of winning and losing and trying to leave behind old addictions like narcissism or abusive behavior, it's often better to be fake, playful, or even contradictory.

Fake It 'til You Make It

"Fake it 'til you make it" is a favorite phrase of almost every recovering addict I know. And yes, sometimes you have to fake it until you make it. Why? Because learning always feels awkward at first, and unlearning old behaviors never feels natural.

When I started dancing. I felt fake. I couldn't even do the moves correctly, let alone do them naturally to music. The first time I tried to do a moonwalk I almost fell over. Now, moonwalking is so natural to me that I don't even think about it.

Because I am autistic, learning how to make small talk was agonizing. Learning how to genuinely listen to people was even more challenging. I knew I needed to listen better in order to succeed as a financial advisor. I felt certain people would dismiss me as being fake when I applied my newfound listening skills.

No, they simply told me, "You're a really good listener."

I remember when I realized stonewalling is a terrible method of dealing with conflict. The first few times I forced myself not to stonewall someone who angered me, I felt like an impostor. As someone who values honesty and being genuine, I felt ridiculous. I thought my obvious inauthenticity would insult the other person.

No, they were just happy I was trying to connect instead of icing them out.

Learning a new behavioral pattern always feels fake. One of my favorite psychologists, Steven Stosny, who works with abusers, says it takes a minimum of five hundred repetitions of non-abusive behavior in stressful situations for an abuser to change. Look, the first four hundred or so repetitions are going to be fake. The abuser has to put on an act at least a few hundred times before there is any hope of permanent change.

Train Your Mind by Having Fun

We are quite capable of training our minds, emotions, and intellect. We can become smarter just like we can become stronger. We can build maturity just like we can build endurance. This is particularly good news for me, given that I am autistic and suffer from some pretty serious mental illnesses.

I want to share two stories about how I've dealt with autism. First, cinema. I knew I couldn't pick up on the social cues that most people could. So I studied classic films like *The Godfather* and truly great TV series like *The Wire*. Those extraordinary productions displayed all the social cues I missed, but in an exaggerated way. Social cues were easier for me to see because the emotional expressions were bigger than in real life, and I could rewatch the movies and scenes. I could go on YouTube for commentary on some of the best scenes, which often explained what was going on with the actors' facial expressions and body language.

I enjoyed this learning. Classic cinema is incredible.

Another example comes from my young adulthood when I was chasing my artistic dreams. I loved the sound and feel of the drums, and I wanted to play. So I did it. But I didn't learn just the basic beats. I learned independence of limb, how to play contrasting rhythms with each hand simultaneously. Learning independence of limb changed the way my right hand and left interact with each other, and it changed my brain chemistry. The left and right sides of my brain now interact differently.

And—this is important—learning how to play the drums was fun.

Studies show that physical exercise appears to keep our brains healthy. But here's an interesting catch. One recent study showed that only voluntary exercise helps the brain.

In other words, if someone is forcing you to exercise, that won't lead to improved brain function. Now I often wonder, *If I am forcing myself to exercise, is that similarly unhelpful to my brain health?*

When I was growing up, many folks believed the brain's structure and function are largely fixed throughout adulthood. I was taught that as we aged, connections in the brain became stuck in place, and then faded or degenerated over time. Those beliefs are no longer dominant, and now it is generally accepted that our brains can change and grow at any age.

I believe I make the most progress when learning is fun. I make the most progress when I'm like a kid, trying out new things. And why wouldn't that be? When we are children, playful beginners, our brains and minds are the most open to change.

And you can probably guess what sorts of things cause the brain to shrink or retreat: Stress. Anxiety. Isolation and depression. A sedentary lifestyle. The usual list.

This is why I'm so suspicious of the notion that we can berate ourselves into positive change. I don't believe in methods of self-improvement that stress people out or isolate them. Whenever I talk about bad habits, I always point out that habits must be replaced with something enjoyable. It has never worked for me to tell myself, *Don't do that! It's bad for you!*

Here are some interesting questions I asked myself when my mind was stuck: *How often do I do things simply because I want to do them? Do I enjoy learning? Is self-improvement fun? Are activities in which I've learned or improved often dismissed by other people as a waste of time, unproductive, or stupid?*

I am an autistic person who became financially independent largely by becoming so good at listening to other people that they were willing to let me manage their money. Thank

God I "wasted" so much time playing the drums and watching the Godfather!

Some of the Simple Self-Help Stuff Works

I'm not a blind fan of self-help because too much of what gets labeled as individual sickness is just a symptom of family sickness. As a result, self-help is sometimes irrelevant and, in the worst cases, contributes to shame. But some of the standard self-help advice does work.

There are seven positive habits I've developed that count as self-help. I hope you will consider the reasoning behind these habits:

1. **I get outside and feel the sun, the wind, and the rain** on my skin. I am an animal, and my brain feels it is part of a tribe or a family. If I am not moving my body, not feeling the elements of nature on my face, and not straining my muscles, then my brain comes to the conclusion that I don't matter to the tribe anymore. My brain may then conclude that it's time for my body to start shutting down. Being that I am a descendant of hunter-gatherers, I also go "hunting" when I go outside, even if I'm just taking a walk. I might play a game of scavenger hunt and try to spot seven people wearing purple shoes, for instance. It keeps my brain and body connected and engaged.

2. **I do not backstab, blame, or complain**, and I don't let others backstab, blame, or complain to me. My brain thinks that if emotions are high then there must be a good reason for it. If I allow people to complain and blame, then my brain concludes that things must be bad.

3. **I do not eat processed food.** My body has concluded that

processed food is essentially poison. My sense of taste has also returned, and now I can taste the poison.

4. **I do not take responsibility for other people's problems**—a primary theme of this book. I cannot make someone else more responsible, and when I take responsibility for their problem, now they have less responsibility for their own problem.

5. **I say yes when I want to say yes**, and I say no when I want to say no., I talk directly to the person I need to talk to. If I allow myself to be passive-aggressive or merely submissive, my brain concludes that I am not a valuable member of the tribe. It concludes that I am not powerful, not lovable, and not capable. This leads to blatant self-sabotage.

6. **I do not allow myself to do busywork** or to become distracted simply for the sake of being distracted. My brain definitely knows how I feel, and it knows when I feel that what I'm doing isn't valuable to anyone. When my brain concludes that my actions are not valuable to other people, my brain also concludes that I am not valuable...period.

7. **I read.** A lot. And this is perhaps the most important of all the self-help habits.

All seven of these habits involve small steps that add up over time—the only way any individual or family makes progress. I don't trust anybody who sells miracles.

The Only Real Progress Is Slow Progress

Unfortunately, I spent most of my life dreaming of the big score, the moment when all my troubles would cease, and I'd be rich, respected, and happy. Back when I was a musician, I ignored my impoverished living situation by daydreaming about the house I'd live in when my band made it big. Even when I became a financial advisor, I imagined how great it would be when I landed that one huge client who would pay me so much it would end all my financial concerns forever.

It never happened.

Nevertheless, without any Hollywood-style miracles or big scores, here I am, in my own house, having achieved financial independence. How did I get here? Well, in large part, I got here through a tedious series of tiny victories.

Progress was slow. And it was mostly invisible to anyone but me. The most important battles I won were internal—forcing myself to pick up the phone, facing one more possible rejection, meeting with a prospect I figured would never become a client, teaching a class only three people signed up for on the off chance one of them might be a good connection, showing up over and over again to events I wasn't excited about, starting uncomfortable conversations with strangers.

This has been true of everything that matters in my life, including recovering from mental illness, changing my own toxic behaviors, learning how to better relate to other people, learning to dance, and learning how to take care of my friends and family. Anytime I've had seemingly miraculous progress, it ended up being an illusion. The illusory progress lasted for maybe a few months, and then I was right back where I started. Miracles make a good fantasy, but the only real progress toward intergenerational health is the slow slog of small victories and tiny celebrations.

If your progress feels like a slow go, maybe you are making more progress than you think.

Back in the bad old days when I worked for the Alliance of American Veterans, I made my living door-hanging plastic bags with attached cards asking for used clothing donations.

Every weekday, my co-workers and I piled into a van and headed out to some suburb. We walked around neighborhoods, hanging bags, avoiding dogs, trying to stay dry in the rain and cool in the sun.

Every day was the same routine. It was a go-nowhere job, and none of us hoped to get promoted. (There was nothing to get promoted to.) Still, there were good days and bad days, depending mostly on the weather. If it was cloudy but not rainy, that was perfect. Summer was OK, until it got too hot. Winters in the Northwest can be difficult. I remember a lot of soggy shoes. A couple of times we even went out in the snow, which was pretty funny because a few workers were Mexican and had never seen snow before.

Anyway, the job was a flat line. It wasn't taking me anywhere, either up or down. But around that flat line were daily or even hourly ups and downs, because the weather here in the Pacific Northwest can change pretty quickly.

Maybe you've never had a go-nowhere job. Even so, there must have been a period of time, and maybe it was positive, like summer vacation, when you were going nowhere. You were just kind of on a plateau. Nevertheless, one day was a little better or worse than the next.

OK, the same daily and hourly ups and downs happen when you are making progress. There is an upward trend, but you have better and worse moments around that trend. These better or worse moments mean that, on any particular day, you might be doing worse than you were months or even years ago.

Progress is never a simple straight line. When you look back, you can see the trend, but from day to day you experience variations around that trend. As a financial advisor, I remind my clients to ignore the day-to-day volatility of the world's markets. Markets go up and down every day, but for an investor only long-term returns matter. There is an important lesson here that applies to every part of life...

One day is not a trend. It's just a day. One experience does not define you. It's just an experience. Look at where you are now compared to where you were six months or six years ago. Look at how much progress you have made. Then remember where this chapter started—with the suggestion to celebrate small victories. It's time to celebrate!

CHAPTER 9

RADICAL RESPONSIBILITY AND INTERGENERATIONAL HEALTH

As your emotional responses change, you will see the world more clearly. True clarity comes when you realize you are 100 percent responsible for your relationship to any other person, and you are 0 percent responsible for anyone's relationship to anyone else. You are also 100 percent responsible for your relationship to any idea, goal, or issue, and 0 percent responsible for anyone else's relationship to anything else. The daily practice of radical responsibility will heal and revitalize your families, organizations, and relationships.

I REMEMBER THE MOMENT I REALIZED I HAD OVER-come my mental illnesses. One morning I looked in the bathroom mirror and saw spiders crawling all over my face. "There's no spiders," I said to myself.

There's no spiders. When I thought that phrase without emotion, in that moment I realized everything had changed.

It wasn't that I stopped hallucinating. It was that the hallucinations no longer affected me emotionally.

And yes, I still hallucinate. I sometimes see things that aren't there. Recently I was walking around Lake Washington at night, which is always when the visions are strongest. I saw a horse walking toward me on the path. The horse was surrounded by all sorts of weird, sparkling lights—fairy lamps, if you will. I thought, *Oh, hallucinations. You are not going to fool me this time. There are no fairies here, and there certainly are no gold, blue, and pink fairy lamps. Enough of this.*

As I kept walking, I noticed something strange. It took about two minutes for me to notice, but the horse was silent. Its hooves weren't making any noise. I kept expecting to hear the *clop, clop, clop* but it wasn't there. Finally, I realized the truth.

No horse was walking toward me at all. Nothing was there.

I maintain that I have overcome my mental illnesses because I have. The key is my lack of emotion. I don't necessarily mean that I can always experience a hallucination with no reaction whatsoever. Sometimes I see things that scare me for an instant, and I feel that immediate sense of fear.

Once when I got in my car, I saw a man dressed in red standing over me right outside the driver's side window. For all intents and purposes, you can just imagine that I saw Satan staring down at me. Of course I felt fear. Then I immediately recognized the emotion and de-escalated in my head.

I was not always so good at de-escalation. I often talk about my lost years, which spanned from age twenty until about age thirty-five. I barely have memories of those years that my mental illness took from me. They are like a black hole. I have many vivid memories from my teenage years, and my recent memories are powerful and clear. But I have few memories of those fifteen years in the middle, and they are weak, diminished, flat, like a faded old photograph.

I have tried to recover those memories, but they don't even feel like mine. They feel like someone else's life. When I think about what went wrong during those lost years, the most disturbing element is the isolation. I often went days without speaking to another human being. That isolation got me stuck in my own head. Isolation fed escalating emotions of rage and numbness, causing them to build into foolish and disturbing actions.

Once when I visited my friend's apartment. I knocked on the door and he was not there. I heard a *v-shaw, v-shaw, v-shaw* sound coming from the apartment above his. I immediately became convinced that whoever lived upstairs had murdered my friend and was sawing the body into pieces.

So I went back to my apartment for a spare key, which my friend had given me in case he ever got locked out. I returned to his place and rummaged through his rooms, trying to find evidence of a struggle or murder. After about fifteen minutes, reality set in.

We lived in a busy, vibrant, crowded area of Capitol Hill in Seattle. The intersections there are always packed with pedestrians, so it was striking that when I walked between our two apartments, the streets were empty. Of course, that's impossible. My mind's creation of those empty streets provides a powerful illustration of how isolation transforms mere hallucinations into something much more disturbing.

See, the first step is that there is a hallucination. The next step is my emotional reaction to the hallucination. The next and most important step is whether or not that emotional reaction escalates. The final step is action. And if anything has become clear to me as I look back on my life, it's that we all make decisions with our emotions.

Once I truly understood that emotions drive my decisions, I could figure out how to break the chain from having a hallucination, to experiencing an emotion, to acting on that emotion. The key was to remember that my emotions can always escalate or de-escalate. I can interrupt the chain. From whatever point I am at, it's always possible to calm the emotional rhythms.

It's much easier for emotions to escalate when I am isolated. When I get isolated, stuck in my own head, I have these intense arguments with people, and I get enraged with them for what they said, but wait... They didn't actually say it. I just imagined it in my head.

Isolation also aggravates addictions. I remember learning about an experiment with rats by which the rats were given a choice between cocaine on one side and food and water on the other. The rats chose cocaine. This was seen as evidence that cocaine is so physically addictive that rats will choose it over survival.

But the rat experiment had a problem. Those rats were in cages. What would happen if the rats were in a rat park, where they had other rats to socialize with, toys to keep them amused, and tunnels to run and hide in? Well, these rats that were not isolated didn't choose cocaine. They chose to live.

Folks, even rats need other rats. I am not a rat. I am a human being. I need other human beings to even know who I am. I need you to reflect back to me who I am.

We Are All Mirrors for One Another

Whether I like it or not, other people tell me who I am, sometimes with words, sometimes with body language, sometimes with their actions. This is why an abusive relationship is so dangerous. The abuser wants to isolate you, so they are your only mirror. At that point, you will believe whatever they show you.

Isolation makes us vulnerable to abusers and con artists. The primary reason some guy emails half his retirement savings to a Nigerian prince isn't that he's stupid. He's isolated. Isolation can be a vicious cycle, in which you spend hours inside your own head, and your self-image becomes more and more distorted. When you suffer from serious mental illnesses like I do, sometimes the biggest con artist is in your own head.

If you are trapped in a downward spiral, you have to get out of your own head. You do that by connecting with others and taking action. The actions do not have to be anything terribly complicated. Attend your friend's performance, listen to someone's story, help a neighbor with a project, visit a lonesome friend. These actions can be small, but the point is to do something another person values.

No matter how mentally ill I am, no matter how depressed, broke, lonely, or unhappy, my actions matter. The way I treat other people matters. Here is the big lie of narcissism—that if you are great enough, if you are strong enough, if you win enough, then you matter. But no. Winning can feel great, but if you've got insincere friends, it can also just make you lonely.

Connection, on the other hand, brings the opportunity for more connection. Just like emotions escalate so easily under conditions of isolation, human connection escalates when you are mentally and spiritually growing.

The Way Out

I crawled out of the black hole of my mental illness slowly but surely. I reached the depths of my illness while I was a musician still fantasizing about some fame and success story that would solve all my problems. I was also working from home for a financial advisory, which turned out to be terrible because it allowed me to go days without talking to anyone. I was better off when I still had my fast-food day job.

Anyway, even during those darkest times, I did one thing right. I showed up. I always showed up to my friends' performances, constantly and consistently. No matter how depressed I was, I showed up. Maybe I didn't talk to anyone. Maybe I didn't even want to be there. Sometimes I went to see bands I didn't like all that much. But I went, and it kept me from falling off the edge.

Then, after a disastrous attempt to live in the Midwest, I moved back to Seattle. I started my own business and joined a network of financial advisors. Most of these advisors were older than I was, and they were more conservative than my other friends in Seattle. It was a second network. So I had all my bohemian musical friends, and I had this group of financial advisors. I joined this group because my business associate, Curtis Erickson, was a part of the group. I communicated with group members mostly online, but still, it was a connection.

As a financial advisor, I soon learned that no one would become my client unless I listened to them, carefully and intently. Maybe I didn't always want to listen, but I learned to do it. This skill served me quite well as I connected with other people, and I learned it only out of self-interest. I just wanted to get clients. Those clients, by the way, became yet another group of friends.

Soon after starting my own business, I joined the Washington Association of Accountants. I joined that group because I had started doing taxes, and I was hoping to find an accountant who would sell me their practice (which I incorrectly believed would be easier than getting a whole new book of clients). So my joining the association was also pure self-interest.

This new group was, again, quite different from my other families—my musician friends or my financial advisor friends. These accountants were what you might expect accountants to be, I'll just say that. And learning from my experiences as a musician, I showed up. I kept going to the monthly meetings. Soon, the members of my local chapter asked me to be a vice president, which was a lot of work. It was work they all valued. Now my participation was not merely self-interested—I cared about the group.

Around that same time, I was making return trips to Tacoma where my father had started his church and my mother had worked for the housing authority. I was volunteering with my parents' friends and associates on issues like education and incarceration. The people I engaged with were younger than I was and were pursuing different tactics than my parents had employed. These young professionals were far more practical and creative than I had expected. As I went back to Tacoma, I remembered why I cared about big issues like prisons.

Eventually, I returned to my old church. That church group was totally different from my musician friends, my financial advisor friends, my accountant friends, and my young activist friends. The church group was all over the place politically, and nearly everyone was older than I was. It got interesting when my church decided to merge with the Cambodian church from whom we rented our space.

In that Khmer church, I had a group of friends who had immigrated from someplace radically different from anything I had ever experienced. Verbal communication was often challenging. I had to learn how to listen and communicate in a whole new way. I had to learn how to interact with a culture I did not understand at all. At first, that meant I often had to fake a connection until I could be around people long enough to figure out how to make a genuine connection.

Then I started dancing, and I joined a hip-hop street dance crew. These were artists, which I was familiar with, but artists from very different backgrounds than the mostly privileged musicians I was acquainted with. I also traveled to dance battles, making connections in other cities with other crews, so I ended up joining several healthy dance families.

Clarity, Connection, and Intergenerational Health

There are still other groups—my extended family, friends from my teenage years, and so on. Today I have more *groups* of friends than I had total *individual* friends during the depths of my depression.

Having so many groups of friends means the reflections of myself that I get back from others are less and less distorted. Let's say a dancer tells me I am disciplined. That may be true, but it is only one opinion, and a biased one. Now if every dancer I know tells me I am disciplined, there is probably some truth to it. But even if they all agree, that doesn't prove much because they are not independent from one another. They share the same bias. They are all in the same dance scene.

If dancers from other cities tell me I am disciplined, that means a little bit more. Still, they only see me from the perspective of dance. But if my congregation, my clients, my network of financial advisors, and other groups tell me I'm disciplined, that opinion is much more trustworthy.

When you go through life isolated or with only one group of friends, it is like trying to figure out how in shape you are by looking through distorted fun house mirrors. You will appear to be out of shape no matter what. And if you get isolated enough, your own mind becomes that distorted fun house mirror. At that point, it becomes hard to imagine that anything can change for the better.

It's all well and good to tell someone, "Just be yourself," or "Be confident, you got this!" or "Just cheer up and look how good you have it." But none of those tired slogans matter to anyone who is stuck in their own head. A person who is genuinely in a bad place mentally does not need slogans. I didn't need miracle cures or catchphrases. I needed to get outside and get connected to real people.

For me, the way out of emotional Hell was to join a series of progressively healthier families. My story is not a story of individual heroism. My families healed me more than I healed myself.

I needed to connect, and I needed to connect with healthy families. Setting boundaries helped to heal a few unhealthy families, and setting boundaries also allowed me to leave the unhealthiest families. And today, the groups that respect my boundaries are the ones into which I pour the most energy.

The combination of connection and boundaries led to clarity, as I realized I am 100 percent responsible for my relationship to anyone else, and 0 percent responsible for anyone's relationship to someone else. Once I was clear, there was no longer a fun house mirror reflecting distorted versions of me.

What Is a Boundary?

I want to discuss something that I was reminded of when I did my boundaries training for prison ministry. A lot of people say "boundaries" when what they mean is "agreements." If I agree with my housemates to certain rules, those rules aren't necessarily boundaries. That doesn't make them bad, obviously. Not everything needs to be a boundary. Rules and agreements are common elements of healthy families.

But rules and agreements don't change relationships. They don't heal sick families. In fact, in sick families, rules and agreements are often just manipulated. Boundaries, however, do change relationships.

So what is a boundary? A boundary is a change to my own behavior. It does not require anyone else to change, and it does not matter how anyone else reacts. A boundary is something *I* refuse to do. A boundary is not something I tell *you* not to do.

For instance, here's a boundary from my prison ministry: I do not accept gifts from prisoners.

This statement is *not* a boundary: "You cannot give me a gift." Now I may very well say that, and I have the right to say it. If an incarcerated person does not realize they aren't allowed to give gifts, then I should say it. But it's not a boundary.

Let's say I have a friend who drives me nuts when he drinks because alcohol turns him into a lunatic. This is a boundary: "I don't hang out with you when you drink." His response doesn't matter, and he is not required to change. Also, notice the use of the phrase, "when you drink." I'm not pretending I can make him quit.

Here is an example of a statement that is not a boundary: "I won't hang out with you if you drink." Why is the word "if" in there? That suggests he needs to change. Well, maybe he does need to change, but I can't change him. I can only change my behavior. Setting boundaries means my behavior changes, and that changes the relationship regardless of his response.

This is an even worse example of a non-boundary: "If you

drink, I'm gonna [insert promise, emotional outburst, or outright threat here]." Here's another terrible example of a non-boundary: "Dude, you need to deal with your drinking." Now, I'm just being controlling.

Remember a boundary is something you choose not to do. A boundary is not telling someone else what they may or may not do.

When communicating boundaries, keep in mind lessons from previous chapters. Focus on the healthiest members of the family and avoid the temptation to focus on problems.

Say I lead an organization, and someone is habitually late to meetings. An unhelpful comment would be something like, "You need to show up on time." A slightly improved statement would be, "If you don't show up on time, we will start without you." That still doesn't communicate a boundary. It sounds more like a threat.

Consider this: "I will start meetings on time, even if you aren't here yet." That statement communicates a boundary, but it can be improved upon because it focuses on the person who is late. The boundary, whether I communicate it or not, is just that I start meetings on time. A boundary doesn't always need to be stated. I just need to do it. But communication is often helpful. The most effective communication of this boundary might go like this: "I start meetings on time because that shows respect for the people who are punctual."

That last statement makes my behavior clear, focuses on the healthiest members of the family, and gives a strong rationale for the boundary.

Boundaries Are Unselfish and Lead to Deeper Connection

When I have some work that needs to be done, but the room in which I'm working is messy, first the room gets cleaned. That's who I am on a day-to-day, minute-to-minute level—someone who prioritizes order.

Many people do not prioritize order and cleanliness, at least not to the extent I do. I have housemates. When I come home to a dirty house, my disgust or irritation is reflected on my face. It is apparent before I even feel it because feelings are just the tail end of emotions. It is apparent before I have time to change my body language or my bearing. So other people know I am angry before I even feel the anger. They know I'm disgusted before disgust even registers in my mind.

Other people are unconsciously aware of my disgust before I am consciously aware of it. They react to my emotional state, and they react before being aware of their own feelings. If we're not careful, such reactions might spiral out of control.

When you are attached to people, environments, or situations that violate your deep values, your disgust, anger, or unhappiness is reflected in your face, voice, and posture before you even feel it. And the people around you can tell. They might resent you for it. They can't hide their resentment, just like you can't conceal your disgust. So you resent them for resenting you.

Setting clear boundaries is unselfish because it breaks this cycle of resentment. When I rent out my house and make it clear which areas are mine and which are common areas, two things happen. First, everyone knows to stay out of my area, which I get to keep as clean as I like. Second, I expect that the common areas will never be as clean as I'd like them to be. I can just accept it, make peace with it, and move on. I own the house and I'm the one who designated those areas as common. So that means they will be messy (by my standards). The potential cycle of resentment ends before it even starts.

It's so uncomfortable hanging out with someone who doesn't really want to be there. It's so frustrating to work on a project with someone who isn't engaged. It's easy to resent someone who says yes to a request but then completes the task half-heartedly. When we want to say no but say yes instead, we make ourselves uncomfortable, frustrated, or resentful. We also make everyone else uncomfortable, frustrated, or resentful!

Saying yes when you want to say no is what I call a "fake yes." Then there are the dishonest maybes. When you say "maybe" despite wanting to say no, it creates uncertainty, hesitancy, and frustration. The other person is left wondering, *Should I keep asking? Should I ask someone else? Should I give up altogether?* They can't figure it out, so they are stuck. Everyone is better off when you say no if that's what you mean.

A genuine "no" is better than a fake "yes" or a dishonest "maybe," partly because a genuine no can lead to a genuine yes. When I say no, it opens up new opportunities. Now, maybe the other person will consider new ideas or at least a new approach. Maybe we can work together to come up with a solution neither of us had considered before. In fact, we might come up with an idea together that is better than any idea either of us had going into the conversation. Even if we can't come up with a better idea, we can at least reach a true compromise. If we both say yes to that compromise after speaking honestly and carefully listening to each other, then that compromise is still a genuine yes.

A genuine "no" can often lead to a genuine "yes" by opening up new conversations and encouraging everyone to say how they really feel. But a fake yes never leads to a genuine yes. It just leads to more fake responses, more dishonesty, then to blaming and complaining, and finally to outright manipulation. It leads to a family that is stuck together.

But what if setting boundaries isn't enough? What if a genuine "no" never leads to a genuine "yes," and instead it only leads to pressure, manipulation, or even violation of the boundary? Or worse, what if people just ignore you when you say no?

If You Want to Leave, That's a Good Enough Reason to Leave

If you want to leave, that's a good enough reason to leave. Actually, if you want to leave, please leave. Leave for the sake of everyone else's happiness if you can't do it for your own sake. And if you have to leave, the hard truth is that you might have to leave before you are ready.

It doesn't matter whether it's a crappy job, a dead-end relationship, or an abusive environment. Leaving is a bummer, it will hurt, and you will anger or disappoint people. But it won't hurt anywhere near as much as you think it will. In fact, your agonizing over whether or not to leave probably hurts far worse than leaving will.

I once dealt with a Hollywood-style villain. I was working with a financial predator who also dabbled in sexual harassment. He felt he had advanced my career, and since he was an extended family member, he apparently thought I should put up with him no matter how disturbing his behavior. Well, I thought differently. I left. I quit working with him and started a new business.

Was leaving hard? It was for a few minutes. It was probably harder for everyone else, especially those who still, to this day, play his game. But the new business I started worked out quite well, largely because I found an excellent mentor. And how did I find him? He had posted a Craigslist ad looking for an accountant/financial advisor to rent an office and learn how to grow a successful practice. So why the heck did I respond to that ad? I was hungry, focused, almost desperate. Why was I so focused? Because I had already quit working with the abusive family member.

The ad also appealed to me because I could tell he and I shared the same investment philosophy. But that wouldn't have mattered if I had been conflicted. If I had still been clinging to that old, awful situation, I would not have been able to commit to a new, healthy business relationship. And looking at it from my associate's perspective, why would he want to work with me if I were still clinging to a financial predator who also happened to be a family member?

Whether in business, romance, or friendship, sticking around in a dead relationship while waiting for something better to come along does not work. In fact, sticking around is exactly what blocks something better from coming along!

When Your Boundaries Are Respected

I have a good friend who kept getting ostracized by his friend groups because of his drunken behavior. But they habitually accepted him back, only to enable that same behavior! They acted as though they had to either reject him completely or else accept all his detrimental habits. And of course, they also set up interventions for him, tried to manipulate his family, and got in physical fights with him over his drunkenness. None of that helped.

It seemed they couldn't imagine setting boundaries with him. I set boundaries. I told him I wouldn't hang out with him when he was drinking. Boy, was he angry. The first time I kicked him out of my car because I could tell he was drunk, he looked utterly shocked. Afterward, he sent angry texts and left enraged phone messages filled with cuss words and insults. He was still pissed off weeks later.

Then I set the boundary again. He realized I was serious.

He was my close friend, and I stayed connected with him. We had a conversation a few months after I set that second boundary. He said, "Lauren, I've never had a friend like you before. You never switched up on me. You care about me, but you don't enable me." That's when our friendship blossomed into something beautiful.

See, I never gave up on him. I never said no to him as a human being, but I absolutely said no to his behavior.

Power and Compassion

You might think saying no is something powerful people do. And yes, the word "no" is a word powerful people use. Maybe you look at yourself and feel you are not powerful. Maybe you think you are not in a position to say no.

But here's the thing about power. Power doesn't just sort of accumulate like money in the bank. Power is either used or it doesn't exist. And using your power makes you more powerful. Power (and powerlessness) are cycles. Power perpetuates itself through action, and powerlessness perpetuates itself through inaction.

To claim your power, you have to use your power. Now you also may have heard that power corrupts. But powerlessness also corrupts. And absolute powerlessness corrupts absolutely. If you exert no power at all, you cannot advocate for your beliefs. You can't stand up for what's right. You have to compromise before the conversation even starts. You might not even be in touch with your own opinions because you are so used to giving preference to the opinions of others.

One of my most grateful clients was in her fifties and struggling to prepare for a retirement that suddenly didn't seem so far off. We talked about several surface issues, which seemed like they ought to be easy to solve. So why did she need my help?

Finally, we got to the real issue. Her daughter was attending an expensive, out-of-state college, even though she had no clear idea what good that particular college would do for her. The daughter wasn't working, and as it turned out, had always attended private schools. Despite her extravagant education, though, she had never shown much academic interest. To be blunt, she was a mediocre student.

The mother, who was divorced, was financing all sorts of things for her daughter—vacations, a nice car, the whole bit. I had only one piece of financial advice: "You need to say no to your daughter."

She looked at me, eyes wide with shock. Then she looked down. "I know," she said.

She emailed me a couple of years later, proud that she had gotten her finances in order, and thanking me profusely for telling her to say no. She said it was the best advice anyone had ever given her, about anything. And her daughter? Well, her daughter is better off. She had no problem becoming independent. She went to a school that made sense for her, and she succeeded there. She also felt better about herself because she was doing well. People are more likely to succeed when they aren't trying to live up to unreasonable expectations.

I learned early on in prison ministry that it's a bad sign when people say, "Oh, you did an amazing job preaching! You are such a great speaker!" When they focus on me and my qualities, that's not good. It means I did a poor job of preaching. They are looking at me as if I have magic powers or am a superhero. If people look up to me too much, they don't see that they can improve.

When I do a good job preaching, people talk about themselves—what they need to change, what they realized, what they are going to do differently. They open up to me about what's going on in their lives and what they've done wrong, which is the first step to getting better.

I don't often give people tips and tactics for dealing with their depression, their history of abuse, or other issues. See, if they go out and find the strategy, then it's theirs. They own it. If I tell them how to get better, then the strategy is mine. They don't own it.

I tell my story, and perhaps they see themselves in that story. I also tell the sorts of stories I share in this book—stories about recovering addicts, healing families, and people who have overcome all manner of obstacles. I tell them what I think is going on with abusive mindsets, intergenerational sickness, and other struggles. But I do not tell them what to do.

When they discover the tactics through their own research, practice, or introspection, then they can claim those tactics wholeheartedly. Because they own those tactics, they want them to succeed, so they believe in them. The tactics are more likely to work, even if on some level they are not optimal.

I don't have to give out tips and tactics, but I do have to live out what I'm preaching. To give them permission to claim their power, I have to claim my power. It is compassionate to claim your power; it is compassionate to say no.

If it's hard for you to say no to someone, think about being compassionate to all the other people who interact with this person. Doesn't this person need to hear the word no and learn to accept it? How is this person going to go through life and its inevitable disappointments, trials, and tragedies if they do not learn to respect other people's boundaries?

The Dark Side of Empathy and Compromise

I used to be way too quick to compromise when I wanted to outright say no. Then a mentor told me a simple parable: "I've got this pair of white shoes that I love. But my wife likes my red shoes better, so we compromise. I wear one white shoe and one red shoe. I look like a clown. Through compromise, we have achieved the worst possible outcome."

If a disagreement matters, rather than compromise, it's better to look for a third solution that is superior to either original option. And if a disagreement doesn't matter so much, then it isn't worth arguing over in the first place. Consistent compromise leads both people into a situation where they feel like they are always giving up some piece of themselves to keep the peace. That often leads to resentment, the opposite of peace. There is, though, an even deeper problem with compromise.

But first, let's talk about empathy. By empathy I mean the ability to understand and share the experience of another. If you are not blind, maybe to a degree you can empathize with someone who became blind because you can close your eyes and try to understand what it's like to experience blindness. But you cannot empathize with someone who was born blind. You have no idea how to even begin understanding their experience. If you pretend you can empathize with someone who was born blind, you are merely projecting.

Similarly, we all have deep values, and by that, I mean deep, biological desires. Trying to empathize with someone who has very different deep values will work about as well as trying to empathize with someone born blind. You can respect the person. You can accept them. You can intellectually realize someone is different from you. You can certainly listen. But when you try to empathize, you are probably just projecting. And that's just about the worst thing you can do in a conflict with someone whose values are drastically different than yours!

There is an even darker side to empathy, though. The strongest kind of empathy happens when we see other people in conflicts. If you are already on one side of the conflict, then you will get defensive when you see someone from your side being attacked. You will share their feelings. And if you act on those feelings, you escalate the conflict. Furthermore, unless you have trained yourself to stay out of other people's conflicts, even when you see a conflict that has nothing to do with you, your instinct is to take one side or the other. And then you empathize.

Let's get back to compromise. In unhealthy families, compromise is a constant reality. The least healthy, most abusive members learn to make outrageous demands that everyone else then has to compromise on. These demands are usually made passive-aggressively, almost as if it is assumed everyone else will go along. Any attempt to set real boundaries will be met with accusations of selfishness and rigidity. "Why do you care only about yourself? Why don't you care about the group?" The sicker the family, the more often compromise is demanded.

Sick families also display the most damaging side of empathy. In stuck families, everyone feels one another's pain, which means no one needs to change, because everyone is so understanding of the supposed causes of hurtful behavior. There is no growth—only rationalizing, excuses, and endless tolerance.

The family remains stuck together, constantly suffering, empathizing, and repeating harmful patterns. The repetition isn't even conscious.

Increase Your Tolerance for Other People's Pain

If you want to set firmer boundaries, if you want to heal, you must increase your tolerance for other people's pain. Those who have learned to be emotional vampires, narcissists, or parasites can see you from a mile away. They can sense that you are someone who feels other people's suffering. You hurt when other people hurt. You can't stand to see folks in agony, and maybe, just maybe, you'd rather be hurting than see someone else in pain.

Simply telling yourself to stop being so empathetic is unlikely to help. You may just feel worse about yourself if you try that. I encourage you to instead prioritize compassion over empathy. And yes, empathy and compassion are two different things. Empathy and love are two different things.

Here's a truth you can verify by reflecting on your life and considering every time you've ever gone through a difficult transformation: People won't change unless they experience the painful symptoms of their behavioral sickness. Suffering spurs change.

Imagine if you never felt the pain of a physical injury. The effects could be fatal. You could develop an infection after getting cut and not even realize it. You might have severe internal bleeding or chronic illnesses you wouldn't even know to treat. You could swallow poison and it wouldn't bother you. One way or the other, you wouldn't live long.

Sometimes pain is not only necessary but also good. If you aren't used to exercise, getting up and moving your body hurts.

When I try to remove someone else's pain, I remove the impetus for them to change their behavior or lifestyle. I also take responsibility for their problems, which means they don't have to. I suffer symptoms that should be theirs.

In controlling relationships in which one partner suffers from chronic pain, gut issues, or anxiety, and the other doesn't, the partner without chronic symptoms is the controlling one. Whether they realize it or not, they are dumping their negative emotions onto their partner. When the controlled partner sets boundaries and heals, now the controlling partner suddenly has to deal with their own emotional burdens.

This is so consistent it's disturbing. I can expect that if one spouse in a marriage starts to heal, the other spouse will display negative symptoms in response. If one business partner uncharacteristically stands up for herself, the other partner will suddenly seem anxious, depressed, or burned out. If one family member demands to be treated with basic respect, suddenly the most controlling family members will lose their cool, lashing out and acting out.

This makes healing seem scary when you begin your journey. When you start to heal as an individual, the symptoms and the family response to those symptoms will intensify at first. The least healthy family members will try to drag you back to your old, sick, stuck role, often by appearing sympathetic, or by focusing on *their* emotional pain.

Controlling behavior doesn't always look like yelling, threats, or physical violence. Controlling behavior can be guilt trips, helplessness, hopelessness, and despair. A controlling person often looks like a victim, and in a sense, they are a victim of intergenerational family sickness. But if you let them control you, they will never heal from that sickness.

In an earlier chapter, I defined narcissism as *the addiction to feeling special or important instead of feeling loved.* Now I'll share my definition of codependency: *the habit of avoiding responsibility by giving your power away to someone else.* Many people think of controlling behavior as being narcissistic. But only about half of all controlling behavior is narcissistic, while the other half is codependent.

Codependent family members try to hold you back by begging for help, accusing you of selfishness, provoking family crises, and playing on your empathy, guilt, and shame. They are often not even aware of how manipulative they are. They just think their life is a never-ending series of catastrophes. But no matter the beliefs or intentions, helplessness is often manipulative. So you can never help a codependent person by enabling their helplessness.

Now maybe you suffer from codependency. No matter how narcissistic they are, your codependency is not their fault or responsibility. You are responsible for changing your behavior. I encourage you to avoid the trap of focusing on the narcissistic or codependent individual. Instead, focus on the narcissistic/codependent dynamic in the relationship or family. The relationship is sicker than any individual.

When you focus on that dynamic, you'll see that it's not just about your personal healing. It's about everyone's healing. If you want to heal yourself or others, you have to increase your tolerance for other people's pain. Sometimes you have to increase your tolerance for your own pain.

Many of us equate healing with resolution. That isn't the way intergenerational healing works. Often, issues are never resolved. Pushing for resolution is not a wise strategy, because it leads people to circle around the same old issues in the hope for a conclusion, a happy ending to the movie, a neat wrapping up of all the major and minor plot points. But that might never happen. We don't resolve family sickness, serious interpersonal conflict, or intergenerational trauma. We outgrow them.

Healing always involves growth. It only sometimes involves resolution. Healing is not always the end of something that happened in the past, but the start of something new that will continue for generations.

Celebrate Your Friends' Success

Studies have shown that a boss who undermines you one day and supports you the next is actually worse than a boss who always undermines you. Wait—why is a boss who is ambivalent or inconsistent even worse than one who is outright toxic? The authors of one study came up with an interesting answer to that question. If a boss is always negative, then the employee never perceives that boss as a form of support. So when the negative behavior continues, well, the employee hasn't lost any support since it didn't exist anyway. Negative behavior from a boss who is sometimes supportive is more threatening because the employee sees a potential loss of support. So the support the boss sometimes gives makes the employee more vulnerable.

Another study reached similar conclusions when looking at coworkers, specifically police officers and their partners. Police officers whose partners always undermined them reported higher levels of stress, had more absences, took longer breaks, and were less committed to their jobs. Of course. No one needs a study to understand that toxic coworkers make you less likely to feel inspired on the job.

However, again, the interesting point is that officers whose partners sometimes undermined them but sometimes supported them reported even higher levels of stress! They had even more absences, were even less committed to the organization, and so on. The officers with ambivalent partners were worse off in every way, than those whose partners were consistently flat-out toxic.

Do you often question whether your friends are genuinely happy to see you succeed? If so, your friends might be worse than toxic. They might be ambivalent. And how about you? Are you genuinely happy when your friends and family members are excited, joyful, or successful?

If your group, family, or relationship suffers from ambivalence, commit to change unilaterally. Support your friends and family and do so unconditionally. Cheer on your friends' successes, even when you are jealous. Supporting and celebrating every member produces the emotional energy groups need to heal, grow, and thrive.

We have to cheer for our friends because most of us seem better at understanding other people's emotional responses than we are at understanding ourselves. This is most obvious during conflicts. I've been asked to mediate several conflicts among my friends and acquaintances. In every case, each person was absolutely spot-on in their interpretation of their opponent's negative body language. They could tell when the other person was being dismissive, angry, arrogant, defensive, self-righteous, petty, condescending, contemptuous, or evasive.

Yet every person was also totally unaware of when they themselves were being dismissive, angry, arrogant, defensive, self-righteous, and so on.

I wish it had not taken me four decades to realize that other people can read my mind. No, they can't read the specifics. They don't know exactly what I want. (When counselors tell you to avoid mind-reading, this is what they mean.) They also might not be able to tell the difference between when I am angry at them versus when I am just angry. But in the long run, people know how I feel about them. This suggests that if I want to change my relationships with people, I need to change how I feel and what I believe about them.

How to Like Other People More

There are a zillion books about how to get other people to like you. That matters in some situations, but it doesn't matter when it comes to intergenerational sickness and health. What's important is for you to like other people. I use and recommend the following four approaches.

1. Use Empathetic "You" Statements

Empathetic "you" statements are ridiculously simple, incredibly powerful, and surprisingly hard to implement. You just repeat what the person said, or you say how they feel.

So for instance, if someone tells you, "I'm having a really hard time in school right now," resist the urge to talk about your own school experience. Instead, say something like, "You are getting stressed out at school right now, huh?"

The person will either agree with your statement and go into more depth...or they will disagree and correct you. Either way they will explain what is happening with more clarity and feeling.

Empathetic "you" statements help put you in the other person's shoes, even if you misunderstand. As you keep applying these statements, you will get to know the person better and better, and you will misunderstand them less and less often. As you identify with the other person, you may find that you like them more and more.

Empathetic "you" statements are particularly useful in conflicts. Say a client is angry with me because I screwed up their tax return. I might say, "You are angry because I messed up your tax return." I make it that simple and direct.

The client might agree, or they might say, "Well, it just seems like you must not care that much about me as a client if you made a mistake like that. I know I don't have as much money as some of your other clients."

I might then say, "OK, you're angry because you feel like I was careless and that I don't pay as much attention to you as I do other clients."

And so on...notice I am not defending myself or being argumentative. I am simply trying to get to the point where I can repeat the angry client's position to *their* complete satisfaction.

If I get it wrong, and they correct me, that's fine. Everyone likes to be right. Everyone likes to win arguments. I just keep making "you" statements until the other person agrees that I've adequately explained back to them how they feel, what they experienced, or what they believe. If this process goes on for long enough, I will get it right.

Every person who has ever had a conflict with me wanted to be heard more than they wanted a result. I have never experienced an exception—not in business, not as a pastor, not in my family, not in my relationships, not among friends.

A side effect of empathetic "you" statements is that other people will like you better too, especially people you don't know well or you have just met. I use these kinds of statements all the time with service workers who seem to be having a rough day, especially if they can do something for me. "You are working really hard," or "You seem to be having a rough time," or "You seem calm on the surface, but..." As the conversation progresses, I avoid using the word "I." And I *never* say any version of, "I know how you feel." I just keep responding with further "you" statements, letting the other person open up. The other person feels like I am actually paying attention to them.

And the reason they feel like I am paying attention to them is because...I am paying attention!

This method might feel strange at first. Most of us have been conditioned to respond to other people with "I" statements. Initially, I tried the method out with people I didn't know well, because I was a little bit suspicious of this new style of communication. I was amazed at how much more I liked other people when using "you" statements, and I was also surprised at how much more they seemed to like me.

2. Listen to Them Tell Their Story

Our conscious brains love stories, just like cats love putting themselves in boxes. (Or at least, that's what the internet tells me about cats.) If you want to like other people more, it's probably going to be necessary to place them inside a story in which you respect or root for their character. But when you ask people to tell their story, often they just tell you about their triumphs or all the great things that have happened to them. This might provoke jealousy.

I would much rather hear about the hardships they've endured, the challenges they have overcome, or the failures they bounced back from. I mean, think about movies, novels, and shows. What are the reasons you like your favorite characters?

Once, a middle-aged acquaintance and I were talking with a mutual colleague. The colleague said to me, "Yes, he is a walking history." It turns out this acquaintance survived the

Khmer Rouge, the communist party in Cambodia in the 1970s. He told of his father's abduction and how it happened so suddenly that his mother couldn't make it home from the fields in time to say goodbye.

He talked about being conscripted into the army at age ten and serving for five years. After the Cambodian Civil War was over, he traveled on foot with his remaining family through field after field, trying to avoid landmines. He eventually got to Thailand and from there managed to immigrate to the United States.

Who do you like better—the middle-aged acquaintance or the man who dodged landmines to bring his family to America?

3. Visualize Yourself in Their Body Looking out at You

"Imagine yourself walking a mile in their shoes" is pretty standard advice. What I'm suggesting is a little more specific and emphasizes that you don't have to be "right." This isn't about being right. As a general rule, the less you care about being right about anything, the easier it is to get along with others. You don't have to understand the other person—you just have to *try* to understand.

I imagine myself in their body, looking out at me. Yes, it is another weird method. As with other methods, I initially used it on people I didn't know because I wasn't sure how it would go over. But it works. It changes my experience of other people and, in some cases, transforms my feelings about them.

If you use this method, you might also learn some things about yourself. They may be unpleasant at first, but the learning process will be worth it.

4. Focus on Their Qualities that You Don't Have

When I say, "focus on their qualities," I mean *tell them*. Say, out loud, what you like about them, specifically pointing out qualities or characteristics you don't possess. I once told a fellow dancer that she was brilliant at marketing. My marketing skills are atrocious. Months later, she said to me, "You know what's funny? Ever since you told me that, I've gotten a lot better at marketing." This is a fantastic side effect of focusing on other people's strengths. You encourage them to become their best selves.

It is so much more effective to learn how to love than it is to try to be loveable. The more I tried to get other people to love me, the more I pushed them away. When I focus on caring about them and seeing them for who they are, they want to get closer.

I also want to mention something subtle that I didn't realize until recently. I often say it's important to not take sides. Well, if I don't listen to *every* member of the family, if I don't at least try to like them, then I am implicitly taking sides. I am ignoring the ones who are not my favorites. That will blow up in my face the moment there is a serious conflict. Not taking sides isn't just a passive principle—it requires daily action.

Radical Responsibility

The concept of responsibility ties together everything that I, as an individual, can do to heal intergenerational sickness. Way back in the first chapter, I provided a definition of family sickness: *trying to control someone's relationship to someone else.* Radical responsibility is the exact opposite of sickness, and it sums up everything I can do to create, maintain, and grow healthy families, organizations, and relationships.

Obviously, no individual can produce intergenerational health alone. But you will contribute to the intergenerational health of your families to the exact extent that you live out the following truths about responsibility:

1. I am 100 percent responsible for my relationship to any person.
2. I am 100 percent responsible for my relationship to any group or family.
3. I am 100 percent responsible for my relationship to my goals, values, ideas, purpose, mission, habits, and problems.
4. I am 0 percent responsible for anyone else's relationship to anyone else.
5. I am 0 percent responsible for anyone else's relationship to any group or family.
6. I am 0 percent responsible for anyone else's relationship to their goals, values, ideas, purpose, mission, habits, and problems.

I encourage you to think, pray, and meditate on these statements. When I say 100 percent, I mean *100 percent*. And when I say 0 percent, I mean *zero*.

The constant, day-to-day, minute-by-minute practice of responsibility transformed me. But it almost didn't feel like I was the one who had changed. It seemed like the world around me was different. Everything was made new, as if I had stepped out of a fog into bright morning sunlight. Or like when the airplane lands, your ears pop and you realize how muddled your hearing was.

I could never have achieved clarity without learning to set good boundaries, and I've often said that setting boundaries with my mother was like defeating the final boss in a video game. When she was moving from her old house to the new apartment, she asked me to haul some things she didn't want the moving company to take. The request, of course, was ridiculous. They are the professionals, not I.

When I said no to her request, I felt like I had conquered some ancient enemy. In hindsight, it seems like such a simple "no." Well, the "no" itself was simple. But saying it to my mother was hard. And saying no to her led me to realize what I had always hidden from myself: I was trying to control my mother.

My grandfather died when I was two years old. So this family story happened before I have conscious memories. Our family had just moved to Atlanta where my father had his first call as a pastor. My mother was pregnant with my sister. She was alone and isolated in our apartment. She was in a new place where she had no friends yet. My father worked all the time, as first-time pastors often do. My mother and I were alone in that apartment.

Then my mother's father died. I don't know how I reacted to that, or rather I don't remember. But I can come up with some pretty good guesses. I believe I tried to save my mother from her grief over her father's sudden death. I also believe I tried to save her from whatever was happening in her relationship with her husband, my father. I believe I felt responsible for my mother's relationship with her father and her husband way back then, at two years old. I tried to save her. In other words, I tried to control her.

Looking back on it, I think I've been trying to control my mother my whole life. But I never saw it that way. I just thought I was being helpful or being a good son. In fact, I would have said that my mother was trying to control me—and maybe she was. But that's not my problem, not my responsibility.

Now that I see how much my relationship with my mother improved after I set clear boundaries, I wish I had not taken so long to stop trying to control my mother's relationship with my father and grandfather. Everyone could have been a lot happier. I can't go back and redo the past, but I hope this story helps someone, somewhere.

If you are always thinking about someone, and you believe they are trying to control you, consider another perspective. After all, you are always thinking about them. Even if they are trying to control you, perhaps the effort is mutual.

True freedom came when I stopped controlling others, because that was the end of my participation in intergenerational sickness. However, I couldn't have gotten there without setting boundaries that prevented others from controlling me. It had to happen at the same time. Hypothetically, it might be possible to stop being controlling toward others even if I'm stuck in unhealthy situations. But it's hard to imagine how that would work. We all get used to our families, so the way others treat us seems normal. And if behavior is seen as normal, it is likely to be repeated.

Your family history, your gifts, and your values are different from mine, so I don't know what your relationships will look like when you take 100 percent responsibility for them. I do know, though, that they won't look normal to you—not at first. Let me offer words of encouragement because the path to intergenerational health is uncomfortable, challenging, and even distressing at first.

When I took 100 percent responsibility for my relationships, I realized I needed to put much more effort into some of them. I needed to reach out and show more appreciation. I told people how much they meant to me and told them frequently. I became a much better listener and made time for my closest friends and family. I helped folks physically, financially, and emotionally.

I thought it would be hard to expend so much energy. It wasn't. It was much harder for me to learn to take zero responsibility for other people's relationships, especially their relationships to their own problems and addictions. But it had to be done. Once I did it, I felt as though a massive load had been lifted off my back. I felt lighter, like I was carrying less weight when I walked.

I don't feel burdened by other people anymore. I see now that it was never a burden for me to take responsibility for my relationships. That yoke is light. The burden was in trying to control, manipulate, or even just worry about other people's relationships to one another. For so long, I mistakenly believed that caring about others is hard. No, loving others is easy. What's hard is trying to save them, because I am no savior.

My Father and My Mother

I would like to conclude this book by returning to the original family triangle: mother, father, and child. I want to thank my father and my mother.

When I started as a pastor, it seemed like everyone wanted me to follow in my father's footsteps, to be a second version of him. I could never do that. But one close friend knew I shouldn't try to be my father's replica. "Your father was charismatic. But sometimes he relied on that charisma. And maybe you will be able to do what he always wanted to do but could not."

My father always wanted to write a book. I don't know that this is the book he'd have written, but I know he loves the stories. He had a humorous take on the line, "Suffering builds character." He always added, "And we sure do have a lot of characters in this church, don't we?" I thank him for teaching me to be a storyteller.

My mother wrote at least one book. Oh, and did I mention that my mother was an English major? She loved to read and talked to me all the time about her favorite authors. I thank her for showing me that reading is joyful and wonder filled.

So thank you to both of my parents for raising me in a house filled with books.

I used to think it was a tragedy that it takes so much effort to write a book, which is so easy to read. Now I see that as a clear example of how health and wisdom can be passed on from generation to generation. When I remember my parents' bookshelves, I imagine this text sitting there next to all those authors we loved. I hope this book is a worthwhile addition.

www.ingramcontent.com/pod-product-compliance
Lightning Source LLC
Chambersburg PA
CBHW031118020426
42333CB00012B/127